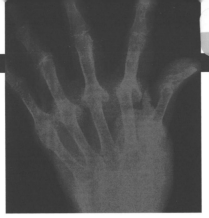

Rheumatoid Arthritis

Epidemiology, Pathogenesis and Treatment

ReMEDICA State of the Art series

ISSN 1472-4626

Also available

Management of Atherosclerotic Carotid Disease

Management of Peripheral Arterial Disease

Forthcoming titles

Management of Inflammatory Bowel Disease

Multiple Myeloma

Published by ReMEDICA Publishing Limited
32-38 Osnaburgh Street, London, NW1 3ND, UK

Tel: +44 20 7388 7677
Fax: +44 20 7388 7678
Email: books@remedica.com
www.remedica.com

© 2001 ReMEDICA Publishing Limited
Publication date January 2001

ISBN 1 901346 16 1

British Library Cataloguing-in-Publication Data
A catalogue record for this book is available from the British Library.

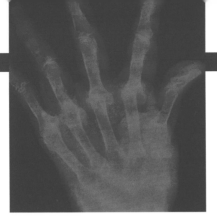

Rheumatoid Arthritis

Epidemiology, Pathogenesis and Treatment

Editor

Larry W Moreland
The University of Alabama at Birmingham
Birmingham, AL, USA

ReMEDICAPUBLISHING

Contributors

Editor

Larry W Moreland
Professor of Medicine
Director, Arthritis Clinical Intervention Program
Director, Pittman General Clinical Research Center
The University of Alabama at Birmingham
1717 6th Avenue, South SRC 068
Birmingham, AL 35294-7201
USA

Authors

Gary S Firestein
Professor of Medicine
Chief, Division of Rheumatology, Allergy
and Immunology
UCSD School of Medicine
9500 Gilman Drive
La Jolla, CA 90932-0656
USA

Sherine E Gabriel
Professor of Medicine and Epidemiology
Department of Health Sciences Research
Mayo Foundation
200 First St. SW
Rochester, MN 55905
USA

Mark C Genovese
Assistant Professor of Medicine
Chief of Clinical Services
Division of Immunology and
Rheumatology
Stanford University School of Medicine
1000 Welch Road Suite #203
Palo Alto, CA 94304
USA

Arthur Kavanaugh
Associate Professor of Medicine
Director, Center for Innovative Therapy
Division of Rheumatology, Allergy,
Immunology
The University of California San Diego
9500 Gilman Drive
La Jolla, CA 92093-0943
USA

Harold E Paulus
Professor of Medicine
UCLA Division of Rheumatology
1000 Veteran Avenue,
Los Angeles CA 90095-1670
USA

William H Robinson
Division of Immunology and
Rheumatology
Stanford University School of Medicine
Stanford, CA 94305
USA

Contents

1

An introduction to the modern management of rheumatoid arthritis

Larry W Moreland

The last few years have witnessed tremendous advances in the treatment of rheumatoid arthritis (RA). New therapies include potentially safer (but not more effective in terms of pain control) cyclooxygenase-2 specific nonsteroidal anti-inflammatory drugs, leflunomide [1-7] and two tumor necrosis factor (TNF) inhibitors, etanercept and infliximab [8-14]. In addition, the first device (Prosorba column) has been approved by the FDA [15].

Although profound clinical improvements have been demonstrated with these new disease-modifying anti-rheumatic drugs (DMARDs) in placebo-controlled trials, few remissions have been documented, and some patients have not shown significant improvement. Thus, the challenge faced by clinicians is how to administer these new therapies—either alone or in combination with currently available DMARDs such as methotrexate, sulfasalazine, hydroxychloroquine, cyclosporine, gold salts and corticosteroids [16-22].

The ultimate goal of RA management is to restore the patient to normal non-RA status, i.e. asymptomatic, with normal physical, social and emotional function and capacity to work, and with structurally and anatomically normal joints. Once achieved, this normalcy should be sustained without further medical intervention, i.e. the patient should have been cured. Although this is the optimal view, this goal can only be achieved at the onset of RA before any irreversible joint damage or cartilage damage has occurred.

Up to three-quarters of RA patients develop evidence of permanent damage (erosion of bone and cartilage) within 3 years of disease initiation. This has led to a growing consensus that RA patients should be treated earlier using the 'best' DMARDs. The consensus has been further validated with recent reports that several DMARDs can slow disease progression, as measured radiographically.

These observations have increased expectations of therapeutic efficacy. With further definition of the genetic and non-genetic factors that contribute to the disease, rheumatologists could realistically strive for remission as a goal for patients with RA. With the Human Genome Project now essentially completed, clinical and basic researchers have the opportunity to define which molecular mechanisms are operative in the initiation, perpetuation and ultimate destructive phases of RA. Moreover, with new targets under investigation, including interleukin-1 (IL-1) inhibitors [23,24] and agents that block co-stimulatory molecules which, in turn, block the signaling between T and B cells, the possibility of inducing tolerance to RA is now closer to reality. With continued advances in our understanding of cytokine biology, new ways of blocking TNF and IL-1 are likely to evolve.

There is general agreement that the inflammation of RA should be controlled as completely as possible, as soon as possible, and that this control should be maintained for as long as possible, consistent with patient safety. The risk of RA management has decreased as rheumatologists have gained more experience using combinations of DMARDs and as increasingly specific and less toxic agents have become available to modify inflammation. Potential benefit has increased with the documentation of disease-controlling anti-rheumatic therapy properties for a number of interventions, and prevention of structural damage will be emphasized in the development of new treatments. This improved therapeutic risk/benefit and the progressive, irreversible nature of RA joint damage justify immediate initiation of DMARD treatment of newly diagnosed RA, and this is rapidly becoming the expected standard of care.

Not since the advent of cortisone has such progress been made in the treatment of RA.

The purpose of this book is to provide rheumatologists—both practicing and in-training—with a concise and up-to-date overview of current concepts in the etiopathogenesis and treatment options for RA.

References

1. Tugwell P, Wells G, Strand V et al. Clinical improvement as reflected in measures of function and health-related quality of life following treatment with leflunomide compared with methotrexate in patients with rheumatoid arthritis: sensitivity and relative efficiency to detect a treatment effect in a twelve-month, placebo-controlled trial. Leflunomide Rheumatoid Arthritis Investigators Group. Arthritis Rheum 2000;43:506–14.

2. Sharp JT, Strand V, Leung H et al. Treatment with leflunomide slows radiographic progression of rheumatoid arthritis: results from three randomized controlled trials of leflunomide in patients with active rheumatoid arthritis. Leflunomide Rheumatoid Arthritis Investigators Group. Arthritis Rheum 2000;43:495–505.

3. Strand V, Tugwell P, Bombardier C et al. Function and health-related quality of life: results from a randomized controlled trial of leflunomide versus methotrexate or placebo in patients with active rheumatoid arthritis. Leflunomide Rheumatoid Arthritis Investigators Group. Arthritis Rheum 1999;42:1870–8.

4. Smolen JS, Kalden JR, Scott DL et al. Efficacy and safety of leflunomide compared with placebo and sulphasalazine in active rheumatoid arthritis: a double-blind, randomised, multicentre trial. European Leflunomide Study Group. Lancet 1999;353:259–66.

5. Kremer JM. Methotrexate and leflunomide: biochemical basis for combination therapy in the treatment of rheumatoid arthritis. Semin Arthritis Rheum 1999;29:14–26.

6. Strand V, Cohen S, Schiff M et al. Treatment of active rheumatoid arthritis with leflunomide compared with placebo and methotrexate. Leflunomide Rheumatoid Arthritis Investigators Group. Arch Intern Med 1999;159:2542–50.

7. Weinblatt ME, Kremer JM, Coblyn JS et al. Pharmacokinetics, safety, and efficacy of combination treatment with methotrexate and leflunomide in patients with active rheumatoid arthritis. Arthritis Rheum 1999;42:1322–8.

8. Elliott MJ, Maini RN, Feldmann M et al. Randomized double-blind comparison of chimeric monoclonal antibody to tumor necrosis factor α (cA2) versus placebo in rheumatoid arthritis. Lancet 1994;344:1105–10.

9. Lipsky PE, van der Heijde DMFM, St Clair EW et al. Infliximab and methotrexate in the treatment of rheumatoid arthritis. N Engl J Med 2000;343:1594–602.

10. Maini R, St. Clair EW, Breedveld F et al. Infliximab (chimeric anti-tumor necrosis factor-α monoclonal antibody) versus placebo in rheumatoid arthritis patients receiving concomitant methotrexate: a randomized phase III trial. Lancet 1999;354:1932–9.

11. Moreland LW, Baumgartner SW, Schiff MH et al. Treatment of rheumatoid arthritis with a recombinant human tumor necrosis factor receptor (p75)-Fc fusion protein. N Engl J Med 1997;337:141–7.

12. Moreland LW, Schiff MH, Baumgartner SW et al. Etanercept therapy in rheumatoid arthritis. Ann Intern Med 1999;130:478–86.

13. Weinblatt ME, Kremer JM, Bankhurst AD et al. A trial of etanercept, a recombinant tumor necrosis factor receptor: Fc fusion protein, in patients with rheumatoid arthritis receiving methotrexate. N Engl J Med 1999;340:253–9.

14. Bathon JM, Martin RW, Fleishmann RM et al. A comparison of etanercept and methotrexate in patients with early rheumatoid arthritis. N Engl J Med 2000;343:1586–93.

15. Felson DT, LaValley MP, Baldassare AR et al. The Prosorba column for treatment of refractory rheumatoid arthritis: a randomized, double-blind, sham-controlled trial. Arthritis Rheum 1999;42:2153–9.

16. Kremer JM. Combination therapy with biologic agents in rheumatoid arthritis: perils and promise. Arthritis Rheum 1998;41:1548–51.

17. Boers M, Verhoeven AC, Markusse HM et al. Randomized comparison of combined step-down prednisolone, methotrexate and sulphasalazine with sulphasalazine alone in early rheumatoid arthritis. Lancet 1997;350:309–18.

18. Mottonen T, Hannonsen P, Leirasalo-Repo M et al. Comparison of combination therapy with single-drug therapy in early rheumatoid arthritis: a randomized trial. Lancet 1999 353:1568–73.

19. Tugwell P, Pincus T, Yocum D et al. Combination therapy with cyclosporine and methotrexate in severe rheumatoid arthritis. N Engl J Med 1995;333:137–41.

20. Tsakonas E, Fitzgerald AA, Fitzcharles MA et al. Consequences of delayed therapy with second-line agents in rheumatoid arthritis: a 3 year followup on the hydroxychloroquine in early rheumatoid arthritis (HERA) study. J Rheumatol 2000;27:623–9.

21. O'Dell JR, Haire CE, Erikson N et al. Treatment of rheumatoid arthritis with methotrexate alone, sulfasalazine, and hydroxychloroquine, or a combination of all three medications. N Engl J Med 1996;334:1287–91.

22. Kirwan JR and the Arthritis and Rheumatism Council Low-Dose Glucocorticoid Study Group. The effect of glucocorticoids on joint destruction in rheumatoid arthritis. N Engl J Med 1995;333:142–6.

23. Campion GV, Lebsack ME, Lookbaugh J et al. Dose-range and dose-frequency study of recombinant human interleukin-1 receptor antagonist in patients with rheumatoid arthritis. Arthritis Rheum 1996;39:1092–101.

24. Bresnihan B, Alvaro-Gracia JM, Cobby M et al. Treatment of rheumatoid arthritis with recombinant human interleukin-1 receptor antagonist. Arthritis Rheum 1998;41:2196–204.

2

The epidemiology of rheumatoid arthritis

Sherine E Gabriel

Epidemiology is the study of the distribution and determinants of disease in human populations[1].

This definition is based on two fundamental assumptions:

1. human disease does not occur at random

2. human disease has causal and preventive factors that can be identified through systematic investigation of different populations, or subgroups of individuals within a population in different places or at different times

Epidemiology studies

Epidemiology includes simple descriptions of the manner in which disease appears in a population (i.e. levels of disease frequency: incidence and prevalence, mortality, trends over time, geographic distributions and clinical characteristics) and studies that describe the role of putative risk factors in disease occurrence.

Incidence studies include all new cases of a specified condition arising in a defined population over a specified time period, while prevalence studies include all cases with the condition who are present in a population at a particular point in time. Prevalence cohorts exclude cases who died or left the population soon after their incidence date, and they include cases arising in different populations who moved into the

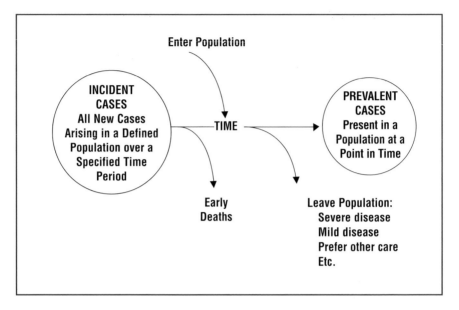

Figure 1. The difference in cases for incidence and prevalence studies (adapted from Fletcher RH, Fletcher SW, Wagner EH, editors. Clinical Epidemiology – The Essentials Vol. 2. Baltimore: Williams & Wilkins, 1988 [1]).

cohort after their incidence date (see Figure 1). Because of this, there is a greater potential for bias to be introduced in prevalence as compared to incidence cohorts.

Epidemiologic studies of risk factors fall into three major categories (see Figure 2):

1. prospective cohort studies

2. retrospective cohort studies

3. case control studies

A prospective cohort study begins with recruitment of subjects who have not experienced the outcome of interest. The subjects are classified according to characteristics that might be related to the outcome of interest, i.e. putative risk

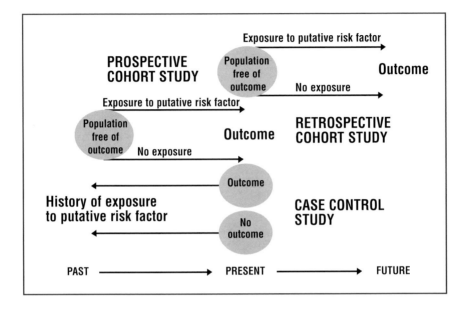

Figure 2. Epidemiologic studies of risk factors.

factors, then observed over time to determine which subjects experience the outcome. This analysis addresses the question of whether subjects exposed to risk factors are more likely to develop the outcome compared to those who were not exposed.

In a retrospective cohort study, subjects having particular characteristics are identified using data from existing records. Data regarding historical exposure to putative risk factors are collected retrospectively, typically by examination of medical records. The subjects are then followed to determine incidence of the outcome of interest. As in a prospective cohort study, retrospective cohort studies compare the frequency of the outcome in exposed compared to unexposed cases.

Two cohorts are assembled in a case control study: one that has the outcome of interest and another that does not. Data regarding exposure to the putative risk factors in both groups are collected retrospectively in order to determine whether subjects with the outcome of interest are more likely to have had a history of exposure, compared to those who are free of the outcome of interest.

Of these study designs, prospective cohort studies have fewer potential biases than the others. However, prospective cohort studies are frequently not feasible, as they require extended follow-up (often 5–10 years, or more) [1-3].

Descriptive epidemiology of rheumatoid arthritis

The most reliable estimates of incidence, prevalence and mortality in rheumatoid arthritis (RA) are those derived from population-based studies. Several of these have been conducted in a variety of geographically and ethnically diverse populations (see Table 1).

Incidence

The Norfolk Arthritis Register (NOAR)

The NOAR is a prospective population-based database, which was established to study new cases of inflammatory arthritis as they occur in the community and to follow them prospectively in order to investigate the natural history of the condition. This data resource was the first primary care-based register of incidence cases of RA ever assembled [4]. One hundred and four subjects who fulfilled the 1987 American College of Rheumatology (ACR) criteria for RA at the time of presentation (1990–1) were identified as newly diagnosed cases of RA. The annual incidence rate per 100,000 population was 35.9 for females and 14.3 for males. RA was rare in men under 45 years of age, but incidence rose steeply with increasing age. In women, the incidence rose up to age 45, plateaued until age 75, and then declined.

In a subsequent report in 1990, the same investigators further explored estimation of the incidence of RA, allowing each criterion to 'carry forward' once it had been satisfied on a single occasion [5]. They showed that if up to 5 years had elapsed between symptom onset and the time at which the criteria were applied cumulatively, the estimates rose by 75% for women (reaching a high of 54.0/100,000) and 93% for men (reaching a high of 24.5/100,000). These estimates more accurately reflect the true incidence of RA. The findings also emphasize the importance of long-term follow-up of patients with undifferentiated polyarthritis and of applying the ACR criteria cumulatively in order to estimate the incidence of RA accurately.

Finland

Numerous studies have been undertaken in Finland describing the epidemiology of RA. Estimates of incidence and prevalence have been derived from several surveys based on computerized data registers covering the entire Finnish population.

A review published in 1998 summarized the results of five national health interviews covering a 30-year period [6]. The incidence of clinically significant RA in these surveys was approximately 29–35.5/100,000 adult population over the study years (1975, 1980, 1985 and 1990). The incidence of clinically significant RA in Finland was estimated at approximately 40/100,000 adult population.

Trends in RA incidence between 1975 and 1990 were also examined [7]. Among the 1321 incident cases identified in the 4 years under examination, the authors noted a rise in the median age at onset (increasing from 50.2–57.8 years) and a simultaneous decline in the age-specific incidence rates in the younger individuals.

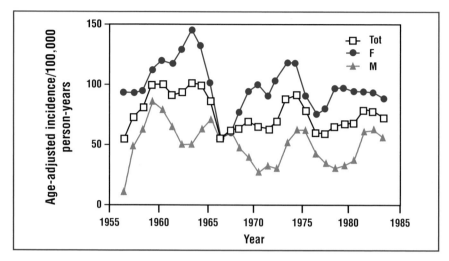

Figure 3. Annual incidence of RA in Rochester, Minnesota: annual incidence per 100,000 population by gender, 1955–1984. Each rate was calculated as a 3-year centered moving average. (From Gabriel SE, Crowson CS, O'Fallon WM. The epidemiology of rheumatoid arthritis in Rochester, MN, 1955–1985. Arthritis Rheum 1999;42(3):415–20 [10].)

The same authors studied the incidence of rheumatoid factor (RF) positive RA and RF negative polyarthritis [8]. They demonstrated a decline of approximately 40% in the number of RF negative RA cases in 1990 compared with the earlier years. This declining trend was statistically significant (p=0.008). In fact, the decline in incidence of approximately 15%, compared with previous study years, was noted to affect, nearly exclusively, RF negative disease.

Rochester, Minnesota

An inception cohort of Rochester residents of ≥35 years of age having RA, as defined by the 1987 ACR criteria for RA [9], was identified. The subjects were first diagnosed between 1st January 1955 and 1st January 1985, and were followed up until 1st January 1995 [10]. The overall age- and sex-adjusted annual incidence of RA within the cohort was 75.3/100,000

(95% confidence intervals [CI]: 68.0–82.5). The incidence in women was approximately double that in men, and increased steadily with age until 85, after which it decreased. Secular trends in the incidence of RA over the entire study period were demonstrated (see Figure 3).

Pima Indians

Incidence cases of RA were identified among a population-based cohort of Pima Indians in Arizona over the period 1966–1990. Among 2894 subjects, 78 incidence cases of RA were identified. The total age- and sex-adjusted incidence rate *per 1,000* population was 8.9 (95% CI: 5.9–11.9) in 1966–1973, 6.2 (95% CI: 3.8–8.6) in 1974–1982 and 3.8 (95% CI: 1.7–5.9) in 1983–1990. The age-adjusted incidence declined by 55% in men (p=0.225) and by 57% in women (p=0.017) after controlling for contraceptive use, estrogen use and pregnancy experience.

Ioannina, Greece

Drosos et al. investigated the records of patients at rheumatology clinics of universities, general hospitals and private clinics in Ioannina, Greece [11]. Cases were identified according to the 1987 ACR criteria for RA and population data were based on the 1991 national census. A total of 428 cases of RA were identified during the study period with annual incidence rates fluctuating between 12–36/100,000.

Summary

A review of the incidence rates from the seven major population-based epidemiologic studies reveals substantial variation across the different studies and across time periods within the studies (see Table 1). Although some of this variation is accounted for by the differing age ranges of the various study populations (e.g. the high incidence rate in the Gabriel study is

Table 1. Incidence of rheumatoid arthritis.

Author	County/Region	Years of study	Age range	Sample size	Annual incidence rate per 100,000
Symmons et al., 1994 [4]	Manchester, UK	1990–1991	15–85+	104	35.9 – F 14.3 – M
Kaipiainen-Seppanen et al., 1996 [8]	Finland	4 (1-year periods) 1975, 1980, 1985 & 1990	16–85+	1321	29.0 – 1975 35.5 – 1980 35.0 – 1985 29.5 – 1990
Gabriel et al., 1999 [10]	Olmsted County, MN, USA	1955–1985	35–85+	425	75.3 – 0 (95% CI: 68.0 – 82.5) 98.1 – F (95% CI: 87.1 – 109.1) 49.7 – M (95% CI: 40.5 – 58.9)
Jacobsson et al., 1994 [19]	Pima Indians, AZ	1966–1990	25–65+	78	1966–73 1974–82 1983–90 8.9 – 0* 6.2 – 0* 3.8 – 0* 11.5 – F* 7.5 – F* 4.9 – F* 5.9 – M* 4.6 – M* 2.7 – M*
Drosos et al., 1997 [11]	Northwest Greece (Ioannina)	1987–1995	16–75+	428	24.0 – 0 36.0 – F 12.0 – M
Dugowson et al., 1991 [66]	Seattle, WA, USA	1987–1990	18–64 (women only)	81	23.9 – F
Uhlig et al., 1998 [65]	Oslo, Norway	1988–1993	20–79	550	25.7 – 0 36.7 – F 13.8 – M

F: female; M: male; O: overall
*Cases per 1000 person-years at risk

Table 2. Prevalence of rheumatoid arthritis.

Author, Publication year	County/Region	Prevalence rate (%)
Kvien et al., 1997 [18]	Oslo, Norway	0.437
Stojanovic et al., 1998 [17]	Belgrade, Yugoslavia	0.69
Cimmino et al., 1998 [16]	Genova, Italy	0.33
Boyer et al., 1998 [15]	Anchorage, AK, USA	0.62–1.78
Jacobsson et al., 1994 [19]	Pima Indians, AZ, USA	0.15–1.0
Aho et al., 1998 [6]	Finland	0.8
Drosos et al., 1997 [11]	Northwest Greece	0.21–0.48
Gabriel et al., 1999 [10]	Olmsted County, MN, USA	1.07

due, in part, to the older age of the study population), these data emphasize the dynamic nature of the epidemiology of RA.

Prevalence

There have been a relatively small number of studies reporting the incidence of RA, and these studies have yielded highly variable results (see Table 1). There are many more studies in the literature that provide estimates of the number of people with current disease (prevalence) in a defined population. While these studies suffer from a number of methodologic limitations [12], the remarkable finding across the data is the uniformity of prevalence figures in developed populations, generally between 0.5–1% of the adult population (see Table 2) [6,10,11,13–19].

Data from the Rochester study demonstrated an overall prevalence of RA on 1st January 1985 of 1.07% (95% CI: 0.94–1.20). The prevalence among women was approximately double that in men; women had a prevalence of 1.37% compared to 0.74% in men [10].

Table 3. Results of rheumatoid arthritis mortality studies.

Author, Publication year	No. of RA cases	Standardized mortality ratio
Monson, et al., 1976 [67*]	570	1.86
Myllykangas-Luosujarvi et al., 1995 [68]	1186	1.37
Isomaki et al., 1975 [69]	122	1.77
Wolfe et al., 1994 [70]	922	2.26
Pincus et al., 1984 [71]	75	1.31
Allebeck et al., 1981 [72*]	84	1.32
Allebeck et al., 1982 [73]	473	2.48
Prior et al., 1984 [23]	199	2.98
Jacobsson et al., 1993 [74*]	79	1.28
Cobb et al., 1953 [20]	137	1.29
van Dam et al., 1961 [75]	231	1.32
Duthie et al., 1964 [76]	75	1.66
Reilly et al., 1990 [77]	63	1.62
Lewis et al., 1980 [78]	46	1.40
Mutru et al., 1985 [79]	352	1.64
Gabriel et al., 1999 [21]	425	1.38

*Population-based studies

Survival

The first mortality study of RA, published by Cobb et al. [20], followed 583 RA patients admitted to the Massachusetts General Hospital for a mean of 9.6 years. The mortality rates among the patients were similar to those among non-RA controls (24.4 deaths/1000 patients/year compared with an expected number of 18.9).

There have been numerous subsequent studies examining mortality in RA, which have consistently demonstrated increased mortality in patients with RA when compared to expected rates in the general population (see Table 3).

Two studies have specifically examined trends in mortality over time. Both concluded that the pattern of excess mortality associated with RA has remained relatively unchanged over the past 2–3 decades [21,22]. The standardized mortality ratios (SMRs) in these studies varied from 1.28–2.98 (see Table 3). These findings suggest that the introduction of new treatments has had little impact to date on RA mortality in the community. However, the effect of these new agents on RA mortality may not be apparent for another 5–10 years.

A number of investigators have examined the underlying causes of this excess mortality [22–25]. Reports suggest an increased risk to RA patients from gastrointestinal, respiratory, cardiovascular, infectious and hematological diseases, as compared to controls. Thus, RA not only takes its toll on functional status and quality of life, but also significantly reduces life expectancy.

Risk factors associated with rheumatoid arthritis

A number of risk factors have been suggested as important contributors to the development or progression of RA. Of these, the best studied have been genetics, infectious agents, smoking and formal education, which are proposed to exacerbate RA, and oral contraceptives, which are proposed to have a protective effect against RA.

Genetics

The familiality of RA has long been recognized [26,27], suggesting that genetic risk factors are important in the etiology of the disease. Genetic studies of RA have focused primarily on the role of the major histocompatibility (MHC) locus. Several investigators have demonstrated important associations between specific human leukocyte antigen (HLA) alleles (e.g. HLA-DR4 and HLA-DR1) and susceptibility to RA [28–30]. There is controversy, however, regarding the mode of inheritance (i.e. recessive versus dominant) [31–33], and the characteristics of the association, e.g. are there specific disease susceptibility loci or do they simply affect disease severity [31,34]?

Irrespective of the mode of inheritance and the role of HLA-associated susceptibility gene(s), the relationship between HLA-DR alleles and RA is insufficient to explain the familiality of the disease [35,36]. The observations of high RA incidence rates, more severe clinical disease and familial aggregation among certain North American Indian populations [19,27,37–41], combined with the unusually low incidence of RA in other populations [11], all lend support to the hypothesis of a genetic predisposition to RA.

A study of the genetic epidemiology of RA identified variables associated with risk for RA in first-degree relatives of probands [41]. These analyses identified gender and age at onset of RA as important risk factors, with relatives of male probands having the greatest cumulative risk.

Complex segregation analyses indicated that a small proportion of all cases of RA may be attributed to a highly penetrant recessive gene. Under this model, the largest proportion of genetic cases of RA would be expected to occur in males affected before the age of 40 years.

Significant heterogeneity in the inheritance of RA and in the distribution of risk for RA among first-degree relatives has been demonstrated. A study published in 1999 examined familial aggregation of RA in the Netherlands and analyzed the effect of proband characteristics on the concordance rates for RA. Cross-sectional hospital-based surveys were used to identify familial RA (i.e. affected sib-pair families). The prevalence for familial RA was estimated at 9.8% and familial aggregation of RA occurring preferentially in large siblings was observed [42]. Probands with familial RA were more often RF positive and had a longer follow-up period. Male gender and history of joint replacements were associated with higher concordance for RA.

Infectious agents

One feature of RA disease occurrence, which might point to an infectious/environmental component, is the evidence of secular trends or disease clusters in time or space. Data from the population-based incidence studies in Rochester demonstrated secular trends in the incidence of RA (see Figure 3) [10].

Using the population-based data resources of the NOAR, Dr Silman and colleagues conducted time-trend and spatial clustering analyses on 687 incident cases of inflammatory joint disease identified between 1st January 1990 and 31st December 1994. These results demonstrated no evidence of a consistent seasonal variation in the onset of disease, i.e. there was no suggestion of any localized 'epidemic' in time. Modest evidence for spatial clustering was demonstrated with non-random distribution observed in one geographic area. There was also no evidence of time or seasonal clustering of these incident cases. However, these investigators did demonstrate some evidence of time-independent spatial clustering within the northwest part of the study area. Unfortunately, the small sample size precluded any definitive conclusions. Further investigation into local factors that might explain this finding is in progress [43].

The possibility of a host-environment interaction has been discussed in detail in a number of review articles [44–47]. Human parvovirus infection has been linked to the occurrence of inflammatory polyarthritis, but its role in the development of RA is less clear. Data from the NOAR, which has the benefit of ascertaining cases close in time to disease onset, showed that only 2.7% of patients with polyarthritis had evidence of recent human parvovirus B19 infection, suggesting that such infection does not explain more than a very small proportion of RA cases [48].

Oral contraceptives

The possibility that oral contraceptives offer a protective effect against the development of RA has been proposed by numerous investigators. Brennan et al. reviewed the 17 studies investigating this association and noted that 11 showed a protective effect and six did not [49]. This group also provided their own results based on 115 incident cases of inflammatory polyarthritis, showing that current oral contraceptive use *does* protect against the development of RA (adjusted odds ratio [OR] = 0.22, 95% CI: 0.06–0.85).

There have been a smaller number of studies, including three case-control and two cohort studies, on the association between postmenopausal estrogen use and RA, again yielding conflicting results. One case-control study by Carette et al. [50] found no effect, while another by Vandenbroucke et al. [51] found a 7-fold reduction in risk among current users. These studies have been criticized for inconsistent inclusion criteria for RA cases; potential recall bias; incomplete evaluation of postmenopausal use of estrogen; and responder bias. The first cohort study by Hernandez-Avila et al. [52] included too few women using estrogen replacement therapy (ERT) to provide a reliable estimate of its effect. A later cohort study by Spector et al. [53] found a relative risk (RR) of 1.62 (95% CI: 0.56–4.74), which reduced toward unity (RR 1.08, 95% CI: 0.3–6.75) after adjustment for potential confounders. A number of limitations exist within this study, including that of protopathic bias, i.e. that self-selection occurs for estrogen therapy at the menopause among those with undiagnosed joint symptoms. Other biases may exist in the ERT cohort in this study as they were selected from a menopause clinic. This study also had extremely low power (20%) to be able to detect a large (50%) reduction in risk, as too few individuals in the study were ever on ERT.

While the bulk of the evidence points to a protective role for estrogens in the etiology of RA, additional research is needed to resolve this controversy.

Smoking

A study assessing the relationship between smoking and the development of RA identified a significant association for the development of RA among male smokers compared to non-smokers (OR = 2.38, 95% CI: 1.45–3.92). Although the risk in women was also elevated, it was not statistically significant (OR = 1.14, 95% CI: 0.80–1.62). The effect in men was stronger for seropositive RA (OR = 4.77, 95% CI: 2.09–10.9) [54].

More recently, Karlson et al. studied the association of cigarette smoking with risk of RA among 377,481 female health professionals in the Women's Health Cohort Study [55]. After adjusting for potential confounders, duration (but not intensity) of smoking was associated with a significantly increased risk of RA (p<0.01). These findings add to the growing body of evidence suggesting that smoking is an independent risk factor in the development of RA [56–58].

Formal education

The risk of self-reported arthritis (a common approach for estimating disease prevalence wherein estimations are based on self-report [quantified using questionnaires/surveys of populations] rather than clinical diagnosis), as well as several other chronic diseases, has been found to be inversely related to the level of formal education attained by subjects [59]. Low levels of formal education have also been associated with increased mortality [60], as well as poor clinical status [60–62], in patients with RA. Notably, in a case control study published in 1996, the risk of RA was unrelated to years of education [63] and no relationship was found between the onset of RA and indicators of socioeconomic deprivation using employment categories as indicators for social class [64]. Thus, while most of the evidence points to low formal education as a risk factor for RA, this finding has not been consistently demonstrated in all studies. Moreover, the mechanism for this possible excess risk is unknown.

Conclusions

Studies of the descriptive epidemiology of RA indicate a population prevalence of 0.5–1% and highly variable annual incidence rates (from 12–1200/100,000), depending on gender, race/ethnicity and calendar-year time period. Secular trends in RA incidence over time have been identified, supporting the hypothesis of a host-environment interaction. However, despite extensive epidemiological research, the etiology of RA remains unknown. Further epidemiological research is essential to further our understanding of RA.

Acknowledgements

The author wishes to acknowledge Ms Deborah Fogarty for her assistance in the preparation of this chapter and Michele Doran, MD for her contribution to the section: Risk factors associated with RA—oral contraceptives.

Reproduced with permission from Rheumatic Disease Clinics of North America, *Rheumatoid Arthritis* 2001 27(2) WB Saunders.

References

1. Fletcher RH, Fletcher SW, Wagner EH, editors. Clinical Epidemiology - the Essentials Vol. 2. Baltimore: Williams & Wilkins, 1988.

2. Sackett D, Haynes R, Tugwell P. Clinical Epidemiology: A Basic Science for Clinical Medicine. Boston, MA: Little, Brown and Company, 1985.

3. Hennekens C, Buring J. In: Mayrent S, editor. Epidemiology in Medicine. Boston, MA: Little, Brown and Company, 1987.

4. Symmons DPM, Barrett EM, Bankhead CR et al. The incidence of rheumatoid arthritis in the United Kingdom: results from the Norfolk Arthritis Register. Br J Rheumatol 1994;33:735–9.

5. Wiles N, Symmons DP, Harrison B et al. Estimating the incidence of rheumatoid arthritis: trying to hit a moving target? Arthritis Rheum 1999;42(7):1339–46.

6. Aho K, Kaipiainen-Seppanen O, Heliovaara M et al. Epidemiology of rheumatoid arthritis in Finland. Semin Arthritis Rheum 1998;27:325–34.

7. Kaipiainen-Seppanen O, Aho K, Isomaki H et al. Shift in the incidence of rheumatoid arthritis toward elderly patients in Finland during 1975–1990. Clin Exp Rheumatol 1996;14:537–42.

8. Kaipiainen-Seppanen O, Aho K, Isomaki H et al. Incidence of rheumatoid arthritis in Finland during 1980–1990. Ann Rheum Dis 1996;55:608–11.

9. Arnett FC, Edworthy SM, Bloch DA et al. The American Rheumatism Association 1987 revised criteria for the classification of rheumatoid arthritis. Arthritis Rheum 1988;31(3):315–24.

10. Gabriel SE, Crowson CS, O'Fallon WM. The epidemiology of rheumatoid arthritis in Rochester, MN, 1955–1985. Arthritis Rheum 1999;42(3):415–20.

11. Drosos AA, Alamanos I, Voulgari PV et al. Epidemiology of adult rheumatoid arthritis in northwest Greece 1987–1995. J Rheumatol 1997;24:2129–33.

12. MacGregor AJ, Silman AJ. A reappraisal of the measurement of disease occurrence in rheumatoid arthritis. J Rheumatol 1992;19:1163–5.

13. Recht L, Brattstrom M, Lithman T. Prevalence, severity and distribution between primary care and referral centres in a defined rural population. Scand J Rheumatol 1989;18:205–12.

14. Mau W, Raspe HH, Wasmus A et al. Prevalence and course of rheumatoid arthritis according to the ARA 1987 criteria in Caucasians. Arthritis Rheum 1991;34(Suppl.):S181.

15. Boyer GS, Benevolenskaya LI, Templin DW et al. Prevalence of rheumatoid arthritis in circumpolar native populations. J Rheumatol 1998;25(1):23–9.

16. Cimmino MA, Parisi M, Moggiana G et al. Prevalence of rheumatoid arthritis in Italy: the Chiavari study. Ann Rheum Dis 1998;57(5):315–8.

17. Stojanovic R, Vlajinac H, Palic-Obradovic D et al. Prevalence of rheumatoid arthritis in Belgrade, Yugoslavia. Br J Rheumatol 1998;37(7):729–32.

18. Kvien TK, Glennas A, Knudsrod OG et al. The prevalence and severity of rheumatoid arthritis in Oslo. Results from a county register and a population survey. Scand J Rheumatol 1997;26(6):412–8.

19. Jacobsson LTH, Hanson RL, Knowler WC et al. Decreasing incidence and prevalence of rheumatoid arthritis in Pima Indians over a twenty-five-year period. Arthritis Rheum 1994;37:1158–65.

20. Cobb S, Anderson F, Bauer W. Length of life and cause of death in rheumatoid arthritis. New Engl J Med 1953;249(14):553–6.

21. Gabriel SE, Crowson CS, O'Fallon WM. Mortality in rheumatoid arthritis: have we made an impact in 4 decades? J Rheumatol 1999;26(12):2529–33.

22. Coste J, Jougla E. Mortality from rheumatoid arthritis in France, 1970–1990. Int J Epidemiol 1994;23:545–52.

23. Prior P, Symmons DPM, Scott DL et al. Cause of death in rheumatoid arthritis. Br J Rheumatol 1984;23(2):92–9.

24. Wallberg-Jonsson S, Ohman ML, Dahlqvist SR. Cardiovascular morbidity and mortality in patients with seropositive rheumatoid arthritis in Northern Sweden. J Rheumatol 1997;24:445–51.

25. Gabriel SE, Crowson CS, O'Fallon WM. Comorbidity in arthritis. J Rheumatol 1999;26(11):2475–9.

26. Hochberg MC. Adult and juvenile rheumatoid arthritis: current epidemiologic concepts. Epidemiol Rev 1981;3:27–44.

27. Deighton CM, Walker DJ. The familial nature of rheumatoid arthritis. Ann Rheum Dis 1991;50(1):62–5.

28. Stastny P. Association of the B-cell alloantigen DRw4 with rheumatoid arthritis. N Engl J Med 1978;298(16):869–71.

29. Gregerson P, Silver J, Winchester R. The shared epitope hypothesis: an approach to understanding the molecular genetics of susceptibility to rheumatoid arthritis. Arthritis Rheum 1987;30:1205–13.

30. Nepom GT, Hansen JA, Nepom BS. The molecular basis for HLA class II associations with rheumatoid arthritis. J Clin Immunol 1987;7(1):1–7.

31. Deighton CM, Cavanagh G, Rigby AS et al. Both inherited HLA-haplotypes are important in the predisposition to rheumatoid arthritis. Br J Rheumatol 1993;32(10):893–8.

32. Yamashita TS, Khan MA, Kushner I. Genetic analysis of families with multiple cases of rheumatoid arthritis. Dis Markers 1986;4(1–2):113–9.

33. Hasstedt S, Cartwright P. PAP: pedigree analysis package. University of Utah Medical Center; 1981. Report No.: Tech rep 13, rev 2.

34. Weyand CM, Hicok KC, Conn DL et al. The influence of HLA-DRB1 genes on disease severity in rheumatoid arthritis [see comments]. Ann Intern Med 1992;117(10):801–6.

35. Hasstedt SJ, Clegg DO, Ingles L et al. HLA-linked rheumatoid arthritis. Am J Hum Genet 1994;55(4):738–46.

36. Rigby AS, Silman AJ, Voelm L et al. Investigating the HLA component in rheumatoid arthritis: an additive (dominant) mode of inheritance is rejected, a recessive mode is preferred. Genet Epidemiol 1991;8(3):153–75.

37. Del Puente A, Knowler WC, Pettitt DJ et al. High incidence and prevalence of rheumatoid arthritis in Pima Indians. Am J Epidemiol 1989;129(6):1170–8.

38. Oen K, Postl B, Chalmers IM et al. Rheumatic diseases in an Inuit population. Arthritis Rheum 1986;29(1):65–74.

39. Hirsch R, Lin JP, Scott WW et al. Rheumatoid arthritis in the Pima Indians: the intersection of epidemiologic, demographic, and genealogic data. Arthritis Rheum 1998;41(8):1464–9.

40. Silman AJ. The genetic epidemiology of rheumatoid arthritis. Clin Exp Rheumatol 1992;10(3):309–12.

41. Lynn AH, Kwoh CK, Venglish CM et al. Genetic epidemiology of rheumatoid arthritis. Am J Hum Genet 1995;57(1):150–9.

42. Barrera P, Radstake TR, Albers JM et al. Familial aggregation of rheumatoid arthritis in the Netherlands: a cross-sectional hospital-based survey. European Consortium on Rheumatoid Arthritis families (ECRAF). Rheumatology (Oxford) 1999;38(5):415–22.

43. Silman A, Bankhead C, Rowlingson B et al. Do new cases of rheumatoid arthritis cluster in time or in space? Int J Epidemiol 1997;26(3):628–34.

44. Silman AJ. Trends in the incidence and severity of rheumatoid arthritis. J Rheumatol 1992;19(Suppl. 32):71–3.

45. Silman AJ. Are there secular trends in the occurrence and severity of rheumatoid arthritis? Scand J Rheumatol 1989;79(Suppl.):25–30.

46. Silman AJ. Epidemiology of rheumatoid arthritis [Review]. APMIS. 1994;102:721–8.

47. Hochberg MC, Spector TD. Epidemiology of rheumatoid arthritis: Update. Epidemiol Rev 1990;12:247–52.

48. Harrison B, Silman A, Barrett E et al. Low frequency of recent parvovirus infection in a population-based cohort of patients with early inflammatory polyarthritis. Ann Rheum Dis 1998;57(6):375–7.

49. Brennan P, Bankhead C, Silman A et al. Oral contraceptives and rheumatoid arthritis: results from a primary care-based incident case-control study. Semin Arthritis Rheum 1997;26:817–23.

50. Carette S, Marcoux S, Gingras S. Postmenopausal hormones and the incidence of rheumatoid arthritis. J Rheumatol 1989;16(7):911–3.

51. Vandenbroucke JP, Witteman JC, Valkenburg HA et al. Noncontraceptive hormones and rheumatoid arthritis in perimenopausal and postmenopausal women. JAMA 1986;255(10):1299–303.

52. Hernandez-Avila M, Liang MH, Willett WC et al. Oral contraceptives, replacement oestrogens and the risk of rheumatoid arthritis. Br J Rheumatol 1989;28(Suppl. 1:31); discussion 42–5.

53. Spector TD, Brennan P, Harris P. Does estrogen replacement therapy protect against rheumatoid arthritis? J Rheumatol 1991;18(10):1473–6.

54. Uhlig T, Hagen KB, Kvien TK. Current tobacco smoking, formal education, and the risk of rheumatoid arthritis. J Rheumatol 1999;26:47–54.

55. Karlson EW, Lee IM, Cook NR et al. A retrospective cohort study of cigarette smoking and risk of rheumatoid arthritis in female health professionals. Arthritis Rheum 1999;42(5):910–7.

56. Karlsen EW, Lee IM, Cook NR. Cigarette smoking and risk of rheumatoid arthritis in the Women's Health Cohort Study [abstract]. Arthritis Rheum 1996;39:S310.

57. Silman AJ, Newman J, MacGregor AJ. Cigarette smoking increases the risk of rheumatoid arthritis. Results from a nationwide study of disease-discordant twins. Arthritis Rheum 1996;39:732–5.

58. Heliovaara M, Aho K, Aromaa A et al. Smoking and risk of rheumatoid arthritis. J Rheumatol 1993;20:1830–5.

59. Pincus T, Callahan LF, Burkhauser RV. Most chronic diseases are reported more frequently by individuals with fewer than 12 years of formal education in the age 18–64 United States population. J Chronic Dis 1987;40:865–74.

60. Pincus T, Callahan LF. Formal education as a marker for increased mortality and morbidity in rheumatoid arthritis. J Chronic Dis 1985;38(12):973–84.

61. Callahan LF, Pincus T. Formal education level as a significant marker of clinical status in rheumatoid arthritis. Arthritis Rheum 1988;31(11):1346–57.

62. Pincus T, Callahan LF. Taking mortality in rheumatoid arthritis seriously — predictive markers, socioeconomic status and comorbidity. J Rheumatol 1986;13(5):841–5.

63. Masi AT, Fecht T, Aldaq JC. History of currently smoking cigarettes, but not years of education correlated with the subsequent development of rheumatoid arthritis: preliminary findings from a community-wide, prospective, nested case-control study [abstract]. Arthritis Rheum 1996;39:S301.

64. Bankhead C, Silman A, Barrett B et al. Incidence of rheumatoid arthritis is not related to indicators of socioeconomic deprivation. J Rheumatol 1996;23:2039–42.

65. Uhlig T, Kvien TK, Glennas A et al. The incidence and severity of rheumatoid arthritis, results from a county register in Oslo, Norway. J Rheumatol 1998;25(6):1078–84.

66. Dugowson CE, Koepsell TD, Voigt LF et al. Rheumatoid arthritis in women. Incidence rates in group health cooperative, Seattle, Washington, 1987–1989. Arthritis Rheum 1991;34:1502–7.

67. Monson RR, Hall AP. Mortality among arthritics. J Chronic Dis 1976;29:459–67.

68. Myllykangas-Luosujarvi RA, Aho K, Isomaki HA. Mortality in rheumatoid arthritis. Semin Arthritis Rheum 1995;25(3):193–202.

69. Isomaki HA, Mutru O, Koota K. Death rate and causes of death in patients with rheumatoid arthritis. Scand J Rheumatol 1975;4(4):205–8.

70. Wolfe F, Mitchell DM, Sibley JT et al. The mortality of rheumatoid arthritis. Arthritis Rheum 1994;37:481–94.

71. Pincus T, Callahan LF, Sale WG et al. Severe functional declines, work disability, and increased mortality in seventy-five rheumatoid arthritis patients studied over nine years. Arthritis Rheum 1984;27(8):864–72.

72. Allebeck P, Ahlbom A, Allander E. Increased mortality among persons with rheumatoid arthritis, but where RA does not appear on death certificate. Eleven-year follow-up of an epidemiological study. Scand J Rheumatol 1981;10(4):301–6.

73. Allebeck P. Increased mortality in rheumatoid arthritis. Scand J Rheumatol 1982;11(2):81–6.

74. Jacobsson LTH, Knowler WC, Pillemer S et al. Rheumatoid arthritis and mortality. A longitudinal study in Pima Indians. Arthritis Rheum 1993;36(8):1045–53.

75. van Dam G, Lezwign A, Bos JG. Death rate in patients with rheumatoid arthritis. Minerva Med 1961;1:161–4.

76. Duthie JJR, Brown PE, Truelove LH et al. Course and prognosis in rheumatoid arthritis. A further report. Ann Rheum Dis 1964;23:193–204.

77. Reilly PA, Cosh JA, Maddison PJ et al. Mortality and survival in rheumatoid arthritis: a 25 year prospective study of 100 patients. Ann Rheum Dis 1990;49(6):363–9.

78. Lewis P, Hazleman BL, Hanka R et al. Cause of death in patients with rheumatoid arthritis with particular reference to azathioprine. Ann Rheum Dis 1980;39(5):457–61.

79. Mutru O, Laakso M, Isomaki H et al. Ten year mortality and causes of death in patients with rheumatoid arthritis. Br Med J 1985;290:1797–9.

3

Pathophysiology and etiology of rheumatoid arthritis

Gary S Firestein

Recent advances in understanding the pathogenesis of rheumatoid arthritis (RA), especially with regard to the role of cytokines, have led to new therapies and revolutionized the approach to targeted drug discovery. Despite these developments, there are still many questions (and many more hypotheses) to explain the etiology of RA as well as the processes that perpetuate inflammation for decades.

The role of genetic background in the susceptibility to and severity of RA

It has become increasingly apparent that an individual's genetic background plays a critical role in the susceptibility to and severity of RA. While some environmental influences clearly contribute, identical twin studies show a 30–50% concordance in the development of RA and confirm a genetic component. In contrast, the incidence in the general population is approximately 1%, and in first-degree relatives of patients it is 2–5%. The genetics of disease transmission is complex, and it appears that many genes (perhaps six or more) can contribute. The genes with the greatest impact lie in the class II major histocompatibility (MHC) locus, which is involved with antigen presentation to T cells. In particular, the RA population is greatly enriched for a specific sequence on the β chains of select HLA-DR haplotypes. This so-called 'susceptibility epitope' is associated with the third hypervariable region of DR β chains, which contains amino acids 70 through 74 (glutamine–leucine–arginine–alanine–alanine—also known as QKRAA) [1].

Although this sequence is primarily found in the DRB1*0401 and DRB1*0404 alleles among American and western European populations, distinct HLA-DR genes associated with other racial and ethnic populations also tend to have the same sequence. The QKRAA motif could also influence disease severity, and the presence of two HLA alleles with this sequence is associated with extra-articular manifestations [2]. The motif is common to most RA patients, but the disease develops in only a small percentage of the population carrying the gene.

While the HLA association with RA might be explained by the ability of the HLA molecules containing the susceptibility motif to bind and present specific arthritogenic peptides, this is not the only possibility [3]. The fact that homozygosity for the QKRAA motif is associated with more severe disease than heterozygosity is not consistent with this hypothesis as there is usually no 'dose response' for HLA molecules and antigen presentation. Most of the residues in the QKRAA cassette actually point away from the antigen binding groove, so specific peptide contact points are minimal; hence, no distinct HLA-binding peptides have been identified in RA patients. Another plausible hypothesis is that the specific RA-associated alleles do not present certain peptides efficiently, thereby permitting arthritogenic pathogens to persist comfortably in the joint without an appropriate T cell response. Finally, the contribution of HLA might actually be due to associations with other genes in the locus, especially the HLA-DQ genes [4].

As noted above, susceptibility to RA is likely to be polygenic. Other genes have not been precisely mapped, but many candidate loci have been identified in animal models such as adjuvant arthritis in rats. In humans, certain immunoglobulin genotypes and genetic differences in the galactosylation of immunoglobulin are apparent. Associations with microsatellite alleles of cytokines have also been evaluated in RA. Certain tumor necrosis factor (TNF) alleles may be independent risk

Table 1. Potential infectious causes of rheumatoid arthritis.

- Viruses

  Parvovirus B19

  Epstein-Barr virus

  Rubella

  Retroviruses

- Bacterial Products

  Heat shock proteins

  CpG DNA sequences

  Bacterial cell walls

- Bacterial Infection

- Mycoplasma Infection

factors for arthritis [5] or related to disease severity [6]. In addition, a polymorphism of the interleukin-1α (IL-1α) gene is associated with RA, and specific IFN-γ intron sequences might contribute to susceptibility or severity. Polymorphisms in the IL-10 promoter associated with high IL-10 production do not appear to be correlated with RA [7].

Etiology of rheumatoid arthritis: potential infectious causes

Although the search for a specific etiologic agent has been intense, a definitive cause of RA has not been discovered. Moreover, the disease is likely to be multifactorial, with genetic background contributing to susceptibility along with exposure to unspecified environmental factors. Infectious agents are, of course, potential inciting pathogens, either by infecting the target organ (i.e. the synovium), eliciting an autoimmune response through molecular mimicry or spread of a normal immune response to innocent 'bystander' antigens. Despite these efforts, no compelling evidence implicates a single organism as the cause (see Table 1).

Mycobacterial and bacterial DNA can be detected in RA synovial tissue samples using sensitive techniques like PCR [8]. However, the bacterial species are non-specific and vary widely from patient to patient. Similar organisms have also been detected in a range of inflammatory arthritides suggesting that the inflamed synovium might act as part of the reticuloendothelial system by trapping bacteria (or their products) in synovial macrophages [9]. Hence, these organisms probably do not have an etiologic role. However, some bacterial DNA sequences (especially those containing CpG motifs) can modulate immune responses and could play a secondary role in synovitis—in fact, direct injection of CpG-containing DNA induces inflammatory arthritis in rats [10].

A viral etiology has long been considered a likely cause of RA. Human T cell lymphotropic virus type I (HTLV-I) infection in the synovium is associated with chronic arthritis, and *in vitro* transduction of synoviocytes with the HTLV-I tax gene leads to increased cell proliferation [11]. Retrovirus-like particles have been observed in some synovial samples [12], and expression of zinc-finger proteins associated with retroviral infections offers some support for this hypothesis. Parvovirus B19 antigens have been identified in RA synovium, and infectious particles can be isolated from synovial tissue cells [13]. However, other studies have not detected B19 genes using PCR and immunohistochemistry techniques [14].

Additional viruses that have been isolated from synovial fluid include rubella and Epstein-Barr virus (EBV) [15]. The latter was implicated in RA several years ago based on the high percentage of patients with antibodies to various EBV-derived antigens. Suppression of EBV infection by lymphocytes from patients with RA is impaired and appears to be related to deficient IFN-γ production [16]. Of interest, lymphocytes from patients with RA proliferate in response to the EBV glycoprotein gp110, which contains the same

QKRAA sequence as the susceptibility epitope on DR β chains. Hence, molecular mimicry could contribute to autoimmunity in susceptible individuals who have been infected with EBV and develop an immune response to gp110. Other proteins, including the *E. coli* DNA J protein, also contain QKRAA and might contribute to an autoimmune response against self-MHC [17].

Synovial pathology and mechanisms of joint destruction

Rheumatoid arthritis is marked by hyperplasia of the synovium, with redundant folds, villous projections into the synovial cavity and tissue edema. Although some studies suggest that the first few weeks of disease are characterized mainly by neutrophilic infiltration, mild synovial intimal lining hyperplasia and endothelial injury, others demonstrate that the classic appearance of rheumatoid synovium is present when symptoms first appear [18]. There appears to be little correlation between the duration and intensity of joint symptoms and synovial histology as even asymptomatic joints in patients with early RA appear similar to those in chronic disease [18]. Joint pain appears to correlate with the amount of IL-8 in the synovium and the extent of macrophage infiltration.

In 'chronic' RA, intimal lining hyperplasia becomes prominent, increasing several-fold from the normal thickness of one to two cell layers. Increased cellularity in the intimal lining is related to:

1. accumulation of fibroblast-like type B synoviocytes (either by local proliferation, defective cell death or transmigration of progenitor cells from the bone marrow directly into the synovium)

2. migration of new macrophage-like type A synoviocytes from bone marrow into the joint via the bloodstream

The extent of macrophage infiltration is a predictor of subsequent joint destruction. The contribution of deficient cell death to synovial hyperplasia is still not precisely known. A large number of cells in the intimal lining contain damaged DNA even though very few cells actually go through the stereotypic apoptosis program [19]. Decreased programmed cell death could be due to abnormalities of various cell cycle regulating genes.

T cells, B cells, macrophages and plasma cells accumulate in the sublining region in established disease. CD4+ T cells represent the majority of these cells (perhaps 50–70% of the total), while macrophages comprise an additional 20%. Although the sublining T cells appear to be relatively quiescent by light microscopy, many express surface antigens that suggest previous activation, like HLA-DR and the adhesion molecule very late antigen-4 (VLA-4). Discrete lymphocyte aggregates can form, especially around blood vessels, although diffuse mononuclear cell infiltration or relatively acellular fibrous tissue have also been described. Evidence for oligoclonality of articular T cells has been conflicting. Many studies have demonstrated a relative increase in certain T cell receptor (TcR) genes in synovium or synovial fluid in RA compared with peripheral blood. However, the patterns vary from patient to patient and it has been difficult to assign specific disease-associated TcR Vβ chains [3].

The rheumatoid synovium also contains increased numbers of blood vessels, although the capillary network is disorganized and the tissue mass outstrips the proliferation of blood vessels. Hence, the synovium is relatively ischemic despite the presence of an extensive microvascular network, and reperfusion injury can induce oxidative damage to chondrocytes in cartilage [20].

The cells that accumulate in the sublining are drawn into the joint as a result of a combination of local chemokine production and the expression of cell adhesion molecules like intercellular adhesion molecule (ICAM), E-selectin and VLA-4 on high-endothelial venules [21]. Although the details of cellular egress are not well-defined, the cells that enter the synovium are likely to be anchored to extracellular matrix proteins like fibronectin using the integrin family of adhesion molecules.

Synovial effusions usually accumulate in patients with active rheumatoid synovitis, and the cellular constituents are distinct from the synovium. Whereas neutrophils are rare in the tissue, they can comprise the majority of cells in synovial fluid. The granulocytes are directed into the joint fluid down a gradient formed by chemotactic factors that include leukotriene B_4, platelet-activating factor, the C5a fragment of complement and C-X-C chemokines like IL-8. Fibroblasts that have presumably been shed from the intimal lining, macrophages and lymphocytes also collect in synovial fluid. Synovial fluid lymphocytes differ from those in the tissue as CD8+ T cells predominate in the effusions compared with CD4+ T cells in synovium.

Cartilage destruction in RA is mediated primarily by pannus, which is the invasive front of rheumatoid tissue. Pannus contains macrophages and primitive mesenchymal cells but very few lymphocytes. Extracellular matrix damage resulting from synovial expansion is caused by several families of enzymes, including serine proteases and cathepsins. Cathepsin K, in particular, has been implicated in the destruction of bone matrix and is produced by osteoclasts at sites of bone erosion. In RA, other cell types, including type B synoviocytes, also express the cathepsin K gene (as well as cathepsin B and L) [22]. Matrix metalloproteinases (MMPs), such as collagenase, stromelysin and gelatinase, are probably the most important mediators of tissue destruction in RA and can degrade virtually all of the major structural proteins in the joint. Although many cells can produce MMPs, fibroblast-like synoviocytes in the intimal lining are the primary source in RA [23]. Expression of these enzymes is regulated by pro-inflammatory cytokines like IL-1 and TNF-α, and their production is greatly increased in the rheumatoid synovium compared with that in osteoarthritis.

Three distinct collagenase genes, each of which has the ability to cleave native type II collagen, are produced in the joint (collagenase-1 by synoviocytes; collagenase-2 by neutrophils; collagenase-3 by synoviocytes and chondrocytes). Stromelysin-1, which has broad substrate specificity and can degrade denatured collagens, fibronectin and proteoglycans, is also abundant. However, the erosive effect of collagen-induced arthritis in knock-out mice that lack the stromelysin gene progresses even in the absence of this enzyme. Recently, a new enzyme called aggrecanase has been cloned and identified in RA joint samples [24]. Aggrecanase is able to cleave aggrecan in hyalin cartilage. MMP inhibitors (called TIMPs, or tissue inhibitors of metalloproteinases) are also produced by RA intimal lining cells although the balance between proteases and inhibitors favors joint destruction in RA. The cytokine milieu in the joint is a key determinant of this balance, and the factors that enhance TIMP production (e.g. TGF-β) tend to suppress MMP expression, while IL-1 and TNF-α increase MMPs but have minimal effect on TIMP.

The inflammatory process in arthritis is regulated by a series of intracellular signal transduction pathways that integrate local inflammatory signals and translate that information into a cellular response [25]. For instance, the NF-κB (nuclear factor-kappa B) pathway coordinately activates an array of genes that direct the inflammatory process. This factor normally resides in the cytoplasm in an inactive form. After cytokine stimulation, it is translocated to the nucleus to enhance transcription of genes like IL-6, IL-8, COX-2 and inducible nitric oxide synthase (iNOS). Animal models of arthritis show that NF-κB is activated in the synovium long before clinical arthritis is detected [26]. In synovial extracts from patients with arthritis, NF-κB binding is much greater in RA than in osteoarthritis, thereby contributing

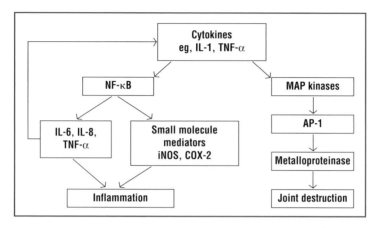

Figure 1. Cytokines and signal transduction in RA. Distinct pathways appear to regulate inflammation and joint destruction in RA (MAP kinases: mitogen-activated protein kinases).

to the abundant production of inflammatory mediators. Another key transcription factor, AP-1, which is a primary regulator of MMP gene expression, is also activated in collagen-induced arthritis in mice. AP-1 binding is increased in RA synovium, in part due to overactivity of c-Jun N-terminal kinase (JNK), which is a key regulator of AP-1 [27]. The combined stimulation of AP-1 and NF-κB pathways in RA synovium contributes to both the inflammatory and destructive components of the disease (see Figure 1).

Rheumatoid factor: the prototypic auto-antibody in rheumatoid arthritis

Rheumatoid factor (RF) is an auto-antibody that binds to the C-γ2 and C-γ3 regions of the Fc portion of IgG. Although its production is no longer thought to be a primary event in RA, RF possesses potent pathogenic importance by virtue of its ability to fix complement and initiate an acute inflammatory cascade. Clinically available tests for RF generally detect only IgM isotypes, even though all isotypes have been identified in patients. Significant titers are also found in patients with immune-mediated diseases, such as systemic lupus erythematosus and dermatomyositis, and in patients with non-rheumatic chronic inflammatory disorders and infections. Rheumatoid factor could also play a normal role in early immune responses by facilitating antigen clearance by macrophages.

Paraproteins in patients with multiple myeloma, Waldenstrom's macroglobulinemia and other plasma cell dyscrasias can also have RF activity. Of note, the specific germline genes that are used to construct paraprotein RF are distinct from those used in RA [28]. Also, the hypervariable regions of RF in RA contain a pattern of somatic mutations suggesting an antigen-driven response, which is not generally true in other conditions [29]. Finally, RF isolated from patients with RA has a much greater affinity for IgG than do paraproteins. These data suggest that, despite the ubiquitous nature of RF, its production in RA is distinctive and related to the pathogenesis of disease.

The interaction between RF and IgG activates complement and initiates an inflammatory cascade that releases C5a and other chemotactic factors. Polymorphonuclear leukocytes can also ingest the RF–IgG–complement complexes and secrete lysosomal enzymes and other products. Complexes of RF are readily detected in the synovium, synovial fluid and extra-articular lesions. Deposits of immunoglobulin, RF and complement have also been identified in the cartilage of rheumatoid joints and can potentially serve as an attractant for the invasive pannus [30].

Altered cellular immunity in rheumatoid arthritis

Immune dysregulation has been observed in the peripheral blood T cells of RA patients. However, these abnormalities can be found in other inflammatory arthropathies and are not specific for RA. Deficient T cell responses in the autologous mixed lymphocyte reaction (AMLR) have also been described in RA [31]. In the AMLR, T cells proliferate and produce cytokines in response to MHC class II antigens expressed on autologous antigen-presenting cells. In RA, T cell proliferation is low in the AMLR compared with normal individuals and can be corrected by blocking endogenous prostaglandin synthesis. The suppressed proliferative response appears to be due to increased sensitivity to prostaglandins rather than enhanced release. In addition, production of cytokines like IFN-γ and IL-2 is low in the RA AMLR.

Proliferative responses are decreased in RA when synovial fluid T cells are stimulated with less specific stimuli, such as anti-CD3 antibody [32]. A variety of suppressive factors in synovial fluid, like IL-1Ra (a natural IL-1 antagonist) and TGF-β, have been implicated in this phenomenon [33]. Synovial fluid lymphocyte proliferation in response to mitogens or recall antigens, such as tetanus toxoid, is also significantly lower than proliferation of peripheral blood T cells. IFN-γ and IL-2 production by synovial fluid T cells *in vitro* is low after stimulation by mitogens. More recent studies of T cell function in RA suggest that T cell receptor signaling might be defective and could contribute to generally deficient responsiveness of T cells [34]. The mechanism of hyporesponsiveness is related to oxidative stress, which leads to deficient phosphorylation of a component of the T cell receptor (LAT, or linker protein of T cells) [35].

The ability of synovial T cells to proliferate in response to specific antigens has also been used to evaluate the role of specific pathogenic antigens. For instance, mycobacterial antigens and the 60 kDa heat shock protein appear to be candidates because lymphocyte proliferation in response to these is greater in cells from rheumatoid effusions than in blood cells. However, this is not specific to RA and is even more prominent in reactive arthritis [36].

Pathogenesis of rheumatoid arthritis: complex and inter-related hypotheses

The pathogenesis of RA is complex—far removed from previous simple notions that strictly implicated self-directed immune responses. At least four major hypotheses have been postulated to explain the rheumatoid process (see Figure 2). To make matters more complicated, these models are not mutually exclusive; several could be operative at any one time, and different combinations might be important at various phases of the disease.

The first model implicates an arthrotropic infectious agent or foreign antigen that leads to synovial inflammation due to an appropriate T cell-directed response in the joint designed to eliminate a pathogen. As noted, evidence for a specific RA agent has been difficult to prove, although patients could be well beyond this stage by the time they are studied.

Second, an autoimmune response directed at joint-specific antigens could help perpetuate synovial inflammation. Type II collagen, proteoglycans, heat shock proteins, cartilage protein gp39 and immunoglobulins are examples of autoantigens that have been implicated. As yet, no single antigen has been identified, and it is possible that 'antigen spread' leads to a pattern of autoimmunity directed at many different antigens within the articular cavity. Immune responses directed against many of these antigens have been demonstrated in the rheumatoid synovium, and local production of RF and anti-type II collagen antibody has been documented. These are likely to represent secondary phenomena that ultimately contribute to synovial inflammation but do not initiate it.

Third, cytokine networks could perpetuate synovitis in a paracrine or autocrine fashion, with adjacent cells in the synovium (especially the intimal lining) producing factors that stimulate each other [37]. Whether this is autonomous is not fully

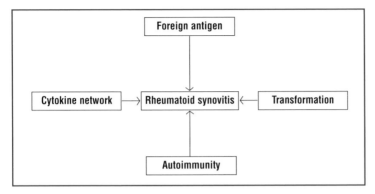

Figure 2. Pathogenesis of RA. Several independent pathways can help perpetuate rheumatoid synovitis.

known, although a relapse of clinical arthritis when treatment of RA with TNF inhibitors is discontinued suggests that an additional stimulus is required.

The fourth hypothesis suggests that rheumatoid synoviocytes assume a partially transformed phenotype after years of exposure to the inflamed synovium and that this leads to autonomous joint destruction.

While the first two mechanisms have been discussed above, the role of cytokines and cell transformation will be further described.

Cytokines

The inflammatory milieu of the joint is dominated by pro-inflammatory factors produced by macrophages and fibroblasts, especially in the synovial intimal lining [38]. These cytokines, which include IL-1, IL-6, TNF-α, granulocyte-macrophage colony-stimulating factor (GM-CSF), IL-15, IL-18 and most members of the chemokine family, have been identified at both the protein and mRNA level (see Figure 3). TNF-α and IL-1 are mainly produced by synovial lining

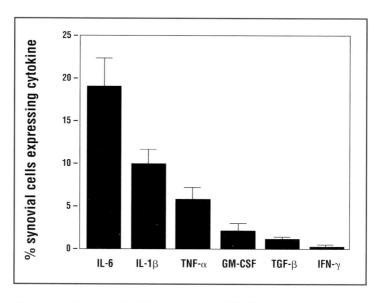

Figure 3. Cytokines in RA. In situ hybridization demonstrated that macrophage and fibroblast cytokines are expressed in a high percentage of cells in the rheumatoid synovium. However, the T cell cytokine IFN-γ is expressed by very few cells. (Adapted from Firestein GS, Alvaro-Gracia JM, Maki R. Quantitative analysis of cytokine gene expression in rheumatoid arthritis. J Immunol 1990;144:3347–53 [38].)

macrophages and are thought to be especially important in light of their ability to induce synoviocyte proliferation, MMP production, iNOS expression and prostaglandin release. In animal models of arthritis, TNF-α is a primary mediator of the inflammatory response while IL-1 increases bone destruction [39]. However, in human disease, it appears that TNF-α inhibition alone can suppress both inflammation and radiographic progression. IL-15 is produced by synovial macrophages and mimics many activities of the T cell-derived growth factor IL-2. IL-15 can participate in the RA cytokine network by virtue of its ability to activate T cells, which subsequently enhances macrophage TNF-α production via antigen-independent mechanisms that require direct cell contact [40].

Table 2. Cytokine profiles of different T cell subsets.		
T cell subset	Activity	Cytokine profile
Th1	Inflammatory	IFN-γ, IL-2
Th2	Anti-inflammatory; allergic	IL-4, IL-5, IL-10
Th0	Variable	Unrestricted

To appreciate the potential role of T cell products in RA, it is important to understand cytokine profiles of key T cell subsets. T helper cells can be divided into groups that tend to produce distinctive cytokine profiles [41]. For instance, T helper type 1 (Th1) cells produce IFN-γ and IL-2 but not IL-4, IL-5 or IL-10. In contrast, T helper type 2 (Th2) cells produce the opposite cytokine profile (see Table 2). A third subset, called Th0, produces an unrestricted cytokine profile. Th1 cells regulate cytotoxicity, inflammatory reactions and delayed-type hypersensitivity. Th2 cells enhance antibody production and isotype switching (especially to IgE and IgG1) and are more prominent in allergic responses. Many cytokines produced by Th2 cells are also immunosuppressive. Th1 overactivity predominates in most animal models of autoimmunity, whereas Th2 cytokines mediate disease suppression.

Relatively low levels of T cell-derived factors have been detected in RA when compared with other human inflammatory diseases like tuberculous pleuritis and chronic tonsillitis [42]. The pattern of cytokines detected in RA suggests that the rheumatoid synovium is biased towards the Th1 phenotype, which is consistent with most animal models of arthritis [43]. T cell clones from RA joints tend to exhibit a Th1 phenotype (although Th2 clones have also been identified). Small amounts of IFN-γ have been detected in RA synovial fluid as well as in the tissue. Its pathogenic role is unclear as treatment of RA patients with pharmacological doses of IFN-γ does not exacerbate the disease and might even be modestly therapeutic. Th2 cytokines (especially IL-4 and IL-13) are virtually absent from the rheumatoid joint. IL-10 which has immunosuppressive properties, has been detected in RA synovium but is primarily produced by intimal lining macrophages. Treatment of animals with Th2 cytokines like IL-4, IL-10 or IL-13 is beneficial in several models of arthritis [44]. Therefore, the relative lack of suppressive Th2 cytokines might represent a deficient immune response which could contribute to the pathogenesis of rheumatoid synovitis. IL-17, a recently described T cell cytokine that mimics IL-1 function, has been detected in RA joints and could synergize with macrophage factors to activate fibroblasts in the pannus [45].

Synoviocyte transformation

The dissociation between inflammation and joint damage in RA suggests that the destructive process might have an independent pathogenesis. This, along with extensive histopathologic descriptions of invasive pannus exhibiting characteristics of neoplastic tissue, has led to the notion that fibroblast-like synoviocytes are 'partially transformed' in RA [46]. Several lines of evidence support this hypothesis, including demonstration of adhesion-independent growth, loss of contact inhibition *in vitro* and expression of many oncogenes. More compelling evidence of permanent alteration or cell imprinting in RA was recently demonstrated [47]. Cultured RA synoviocytes co-implanted with cartilage explants into mice with severe combined immunodeficiency disease (SCID) invade the cartilage matrix, whereas osteoarthritis synoviocytes and normal dermal fibroblasts do not. The mechanism of this process remains undefined, although production of cytokines like IL-1 and IL-10 (but surprisingly not TNF-α) appears to contribute [48]. On the other hand, if the p53 tumor suppressor function is blocked, then even normal synoviocytes invade the cartilage matrix. Despite these findings, RA synoviocytes are not fully transformed as they are not immortalized and eventually become senescent *in vitro*.

One mechanism for permanently altering cell function could be through the introduction of somatic mutations. The synovial microenvironment is highly toxic in RA and is rife with potentially mutagenic reactive oxygen and nitrogen [49]. Indeed, somatic mutations in various genes have been identified in RA cells, including the p53 tumor suppressor gene, H-ras and HGPRT [50-52]. Although these mutations do not cause RA (rather they appear to be the result of inflammation), they might alter the natural history of the disease by enhancing invasiveness and joint destruction. The functional relevance of these mutations in the perpetuation of RA remains to be determined.

Conclusions

As the complex rheumatoid arthritis process has been gradually dissected, our understanding of disease initiation and perpetuation has become increasingly sophisticated. The simplistic view that mere elimination of T cells is the primary therapeutic goal has been replaced by models recognizing the complex and inter-related mechanisms that contribute to a disease process that can extend over many decades. Systematic exploration of cytokine regulation ultimately led to the discovery that TNF inhibition has therapeutic benefit in RA. Current studies are likely to identify new targets, leading to novel treatments.

References

1. Nepom GT, Byers P, Seyfried C et al. HLA genes associated with rheumatoid arthritis: identification of susceptibility alleles using specific oligonucleotide probes. Arthritis Rheum 1989;32:15–21.

2. Weyand CM, Hicok KC, Conn DL et al. The influence of HLA-DRB1 genes on disease severity in rheumatoid arthritis. Ann Intern Med 1992;117:801–6.

3. Fox DA. The role of T cells in the immunopathogenesis of rheumatoid arthritis: new perspectives. Arthritis Rheum 1997;40:598–609.

4. Das P, Bradley DS, Geluk A et al. An HLA-DRB1*0402 derived peptide (HV3 65-79) prevents collagen-induced arthritis in HLA-DQ8 transgenic mice. Hum Immunol 1999;60:575–82.

5. Moxley G, Meyer J, Singh R et al. Microsatellite alleles of tumor necrosis factor show linkage disequilibrium with shared epitope DRB1 alleles and DQB1 [abstract]. Arthritis Rheum 1996;39(Suppl.):S122.

6. Verweij CL. Tumour necrosis factor gene polymorphisms as severity markers in rheumatoid arthritis. Ann Rheum Dis 1999;58(Suppl. 1):I20–6.

7. Coakley G, Mok CC, Hajeer AH et al. Interleukin-10 promoter polymorphisms in rheumatoid arthritis and Felty's syndrome. Br J Rheumatol 1998;37:988–91.

8. van der Heijden IM, Wilbrink B, Schouls LM et al. Detection of mycobacteria in joint samples from patients with arthritis using a genus-specific polymerase chain reaction and sequence analysis. Rheumatology (Oxford) 1999;38:547–53.

9. Wilbrink B, van der Heijden IM, Schouls LM et al. Detection of bacterial DNA in joint samples from patients with undifferentiated arthritis and reactive arthritis, using polymerase chain reaction with universal 16S ribosomal RNA primers. Arthritis Rheum 1998;41:535–43.

10. Deng GM, Nilsson IM, Verdrengh M et al. Intra-articularly localized bacterial DNA containing CpG motifs induces arthritis. Nat Med 1999;5:702–5.

11. Nakajima T, Aono H, Hasunuma T et al. Overgrowth of human synovial cells driven by the human T cell leukemia virus type I tax gene. J Clin Invest 1993;92:186–93.

12. Stransky G, Vernon J, Aicher WK et al. Virus-like particles in synovial fluids from patients with rheumatoid arthritis. Br J Rheumatol 1993;32:1044–8.

13. Takahashi Y, Murai C, Shibata S et al. Human parvovirus B19 as a causative agent for rheumatoid arthritis. Proc Natl Acad Sci USA 1998;95:8227–32.

14. Harrison B, Silman A, Barrett E et al. Low frequency of recent parvovirus infection in a population-based cohort of patients with early inflammatory polyarthritis. Ann Rheum Dis 1998;57:375–7.

15. Depper JM, Bluestein HG, Zvaifler NJ. Impaired regulation of Epstein-Barr virus-induced lymphocyte proliferation in rheumatoid arthritis is due to a T cell defect. J Immunol 1981;127:1899–902.

16. Hasler F, Bluestein HG, Zvaifler NJ et al. Analysis of the defects responsible for the impaired regulation of Epstein-Barr virus-induced B cell proliferation by rheumatoid arthritis lymphocytes: I. Diminished gamma interferon production in response to autologous stimulation. J Exp Med 1983;157:173–88.

17. Auger I, Roudier J. A function for the QKRAA amino acid motif: mediating binding of DnaJ to DnaK. Implications for the association of rheumatoid arthritis with HLA-DR4. J Clin Invest 1997;99:1818–22.

18. Tak PP, Smeets TJ, Daha MR et al. Analysis of the synovial cell infiltrate in early rheumatoid synovial tissue in relation to local disease activity. Arthritis Rheum 1997;40:217–25.

19. Firestein GS, Yeo M, Zvaifler NJ. Apoptosis in rheumatoid arthritis synovium. J Clin Invest 1995;96:1631–8.

20. Mapp PI, Grootveld MC, Blake DR. Hypoxia, oxidative stress and rheumatoid arthritis. Br Med Bull 1995;51:419–36.

21. Cronstein BN. Adhesion molecules in the pathogenesis of rheumatoid arthritis. Curr Opin Rheumatol 1994;6:300–4.

22. Hummel KM, Petrow PK, Franz JK et al. Cysteine proteinase cathepsin K mRNA is expressed in synovium of patients with rheumatoid arthritis and is detected at sites of synovial bone destruction. J Rheumatol 1998;25:1887–94.

23. Firestein GS, Paine MM, Littman BH. Gene expression (collagenase, tissue inhibitor of metalloproteinases, complement, and HLA-DR) in rheumatoid arthritis and osteoarthritis synovium. Quantitative analysis and effect of intraarticular corticosteroids. Arthritis Rheum 1991;34:1094–105.

24. Abbaszade I, Liu RQ, Yang F et al. Cloning and characterization of ADAMTS11, an aggrecanase from the ADAMTS family. J Biol Chem 1999;274:23443–50.

25. Firestein GS, Manning AM. Signal transduction and transcription factors in rheumatic diseases. Arthritis Rheum 1999;42:609–21.

26. Han Z, Boyle DL, Manning AM et al. AP-1 and NF-κB regulation in rheumatoid arthritis and murine collagen-induced arthritis. Autoimmunity 1998;28:197–208.

27. Han Z, Boyle DL, Aupperle KR et al. Jun N-terminal kinase in rheumatoid arthritis. J Pharmacol Exp Ther 1999;291:124–30.

28. Fong S, Chen PP, Gilbertson TA et al. Structural similarities in the kappa light chains of human rheumatoid factor paraproteins and serum immunoglobulins bearing a cross-reactive idiotype. J Immunol 1985;135:1955–60.

29. Moyes SP, Brown CM, Scott BB et al. Analysis of V kappa genes in rheumatoid arthritis (RA) synovial B lymphocytes provides evidence for both polyclonal activation and antigen-driven selection. Clin Exp Immunol 1996;105:89–98.

30. Mannik M, Person RE. Deep penetration of antibodies into the articular cartilage of patients with rheumatoid arthritis. Rheumatol Int 1994;14:95–102.

31. Pope RM, McChesney L, Talal N et al. Characterization of the defective autologous mixed lymphocyte response in rheumatoid arthritis. Arthritis Rheum 1984;27:1234–44.

32. Lotz M, Tsoukas CD, Robinson CA et al. Basis for defective responses of rheumatoid arthritis synovial fluid lymphocytes to anti-CD3 (T3) antibodies. J Clin Invest 1986;78:713–21.

33. Wahl SM, Allen JB, Wong HL et al. Antagonistic and agonistic effects of transforming growth factor-beta and IL-1 in rheumatoid synovium. J Immunol 1990;145:2514–9.

34. Maurice MM, Lankester AC, Bezemer AC et al. Defective TCR-mediated signaling in synovial T cells in rheumatoid arthritis. J Immunol 1997;159:2973–8.

35. Gringhuis SI, Leow A, Papendrecht-Van Der Voort EA et al. Displacement of linker for activation of T cells from the plasma membrane due to redox balance alterations results in hyporesponsiveness of synovial fluid T lymphocytes in rheumatoid arthritis. J Immunol 2000;164:2170–9.

36. Gaston JS, Life PF, Bailey LC et al. In vitro responses to a 65-kilodalton mycobacterial protein by synovial T cells from inflammatory arthritis patients. J Immunol 1989;143:2494–500.

37. Firestein GS, Zvaifler NJ. How important are T cells in chronic rheumatoid synovitis? Arthritis Rheum 1990;33:768–73.

38. Firestein GS, Alvaro-Gracia JM, Maki R. Quantitative analysis of cytokine gene expression in rheumatoid arthritis. J Immunol 1990;144:3347–53.

39. van den Berg WB, Joosten LA, van de Loo FA. TNF alpha and IL-1 beta are separate targets in chronic arthritis. Clin Exp Rheumatol 1999;17(Suppl. 18):S105–14.

40. McInnes IB, Leung BP, Sturrock RD et al. Interleukin-15 mediates T cell-dependent regulation of tumor necrosis factor-alpha production in rheumatoid arthritis. Nat Med 1997;3:189–95.

41. Mosmann TR, Sad S. The expanding universe of T-cell subsets: Th1, Th2 and more. Immunol Today 1996;17:138–46.

42. Miossec P, Navillat M, Dupuy d'Angeac A et al. Low levels of interleukin-4 and high levels of transforming growth factor beta in rheumatoid arthritis. Arthritis Rheum 1990;33:1180–7.

43. Kotake S, Schumacher HR Jr, Yarboro CH. In vivo gene expression of type 1 and type 2 cytokines in synovial tissues from patients in early stages of rheumatoid, reactive, and undifferentiated arthritis. Proc Assoc Am Physicians 1997;109:286–301.

44. Firestein GS. Novel therapeutic strategies involving animals, arthritis, and apoptosis. Curr Opin Rheumatol 1998;10:236–41.

45. Chabaud M, Durand JM, Buchs N et al. Human interleukin-17: a T cell-derived

proinflammatory cytokine produced by the rheumatoid synovium. Arthritis Rheum 1999;42:963–70.

46. Firestein GS. Invasive fibroblast-like synoviocytes in rheumatoid arthritis: passive responders or transformed aggressors? Arthritis Rheum 1996;39:1781–90.

47. Muller-Ladner U, Kriegsmann J, Franklin BN et al. Synovial fibroblasts of patients with rheumatoid arthritis attach to and invade normal human cartilage when engrafted into SCID mice. Am J Pathol 1996;149:1607–15.

48. Muller-Ladner U, Evans CH, Franklin BN et al. Gene transfer of cytokine inhibitors into human synovial fibroblasts in the SCID mouse model. Arthritis Rheum 1999;42:490–7.

49. Tak PP, Zvaifler NJ, Green DR et al. Rheumatoid arthritis and p53: how oxidative stress might alter the course of inflammatory diseases. Immunol Today 2000;21:78–82.

50. Firestein GS, Echeverri F, Yeo M et al. Somatic mutations in the p53 tumor suppressor gene in rheumatoid arthritis synovium. Proc Natl Acad Sci USA 1997;94:10895–900.

51. Cannons JL, Karsh J, Birnboim HC et al. HPRT-mutant T cells in the peripheral blood and synovial tissue of patients with rheumatoid arthritis. Arthritis Rheum 1998;41:1772–82.

52. Roivainen A, Jalava J, Pirila L et al. H-ras oncogene point mutations in arthritic synovium. Arthritis Rheum 1997;40:1636–43.

4

Current therapeutic options: non-biologic agents

Harold E Paulus

Rheumatoid arthritis (RA) can afflict a person at any age and usually persists for the remainder of the patient's life. The specific aims of its management vary among individual patients, depending on the aggressiveness of their symptoms, their stage of life and RA's impact on them on a day-to-day basis. Accepting that tissue destruction and loss of function are due to persistent and misdirected inflammation, then prolonged complete control of the inflammatory process is fundamental in the management of patients with RA. Therapeutic options include: analgesics and nonsteroidal anti-inflammatory drugs (NSAIDs); disease-modifying anti-rheumatic drugs (DMARDs) including biological agents; corticosteroids; and physical interventions such as rest, surgery, physical and occupational therapy [1].

Modern treatment strategy for rheumatoid arthritis

The traditional pyramid approach to RA therapy—the concept of months or years of symptomatic therapy while waiting for a spontaneous remission, before starting a DMARD—is now considered counterproductive. Rheumatologists today usually institute a DMARD or DMARDs as soon as the diagnosis of RA is confirmed.

In addition to significant morbidity (see Table 1), life expectancy of patients with aggressive synovitis may be shortened by 10–15 years [2,3]. To prevent such outcomes, early control of inflammation and the disease itself is critical. Several studies have revealed that DMARD therapy early in the course of RA

Table 1. Impact of rheumatoid arthritis.	
Most patients develop radiographically evident joint damage	0–2 years
50% of maximal radiological damage is observed	Within 6 years
50% become disabled	Within 5 years
90% become disabled	Within 30 years

slows disease progression more effectively than delayed DMARD use [4,5]. In addition, the benefit of DMARDs is indicated by the increased frequency of exacerbations when they are discontinued in patients who are in remission [6]. Fortunately, controlled clinical trials have demonstrated that measurable radiographic progression of joint damage can be decreased by DMARDs: leflunomide, methotrexate, sulfasalazine [7] and infliximab [8] were compared to placebo in patients with well-established RA of 5–15 years' duration; and etanercept [9] and leflunomide [7] were compared to methotrexate in patients with relatively early RA of 1–5 years' duration. In these studies, improvement of signs, symptoms and function also occurred.

Nonsteroidal anti-inflammatory drugs (NSAIDs)

NSAIDs reduce the signs and symptoms of inflammation, but do not eliminate the underlying cause. Their effects on pain, swelling, heat, erythema and loss of function begin promptly after their absorption into the blood and become fully evident within a few weeks. Drug withdrawal is quickly followed by an exacerbation. Joint damage continues during the administration of NSAIDs to RA patients.

Cyclooxygenase-1 and cyclooxygenase-2

Various hypotheses have been advanced to explain the actions of NSAIDs. In 1971, Vane proposed that the major therapeutic and toxic effects of NSAIDs might be accounted

---

Table 2. The main properties of COX-1 and COX-2.

COX-1   Present in many tissues

Responsible for the physiologic production of homeostatic and cytoprotective prostanoids in the gastric mucosa, endothelium, platelets and kidney

Its inhibition is linked to many of the familiar adverse effects of NSAIDs

COX-2   Induced during inflammation and tissue repair

Pro-inflammatory stimuli induce production in leukocytes, vascular smooth muscle cells, human rheumatoid synoviocytes and brain neurons

Induction in the brain is associated with neurogenic pain and fever

Physiologically involved in the timing of ovulation and implantation of the blastocyst in the uterine wall

Physiologically involved in bone remodeling

Induced in renal macula densa and medullary interstitial cells during sodium restriction [12]

Expressed in the podocytes of the human glomerulus. Specific COX-2 inhibitors induce transient sodium retention without altering glomerular filtration rate [12]

Expressed in endothelial cells of renal arteries and veins, and upregulated by inhibitors of angiotensin converting enzyme

---

for by their ability to suppress the synthesis of prostaglandins by inhibiting the enzyme cyclooxygenase [10]. Cyclooxygenase exists in two forms: cyclooxygenase-1 and cyclooxygenase-2 (COX-1 and COX-2) [11]. Their main properties are summarized in Table 2.

Available nonsteroidal anti-inflammatory drugs

To a considerable extent, the clinical properties and side effect profiles of NSAIDs are explained by their suppression of COX-1 and COX-2. Effective doses of all NSAIDs inhibit COX-2 (see Table 3). Most NSAIDs inhibit COX-1 more efficiently than COX-2. COX-1 preferential NSAIDs include: aspirin, indomethacin, ibuprofen, naproxen and piroxicam. Non-acetylated salicylates and diclofenac are approximately equal inhibitors of COX-1 and COX-2. Etodolac and meloxicam are COX-2 preferential by a ratio

Table 3. Clinical properties and side effect profiles of some NSAIDs.

(all NSAIDs suppress COX-2)

	Dose-range (mg/day)	Half-life (hours)	GI adverse effects Symptoms	GI adverse effects Ulcers, bleeds, perforations	Comments
COX-1 preferential					
Aspirin	1000–6000	4–15	+++	2–4%/year	Overdose lethal, platelet anticoagulant
Indomethacin	50–200	3–11	+++	2–4%/year	
Ibuprofen	1200–3000	2	++ to +++	2–4%/year	
Naproxen	250–1500	13	++ to +++	2–4%/year	
Piroxicam	20	30–86	+++	2–4%/year	
COX-1/COX-2 equal					
Non-acetylated salicylates	1500–5000	4–15	+ to ++	Uncertain	Overdose lethal
Diclofenac	75–150	1–2	++	2–4%/year	Increased liver toxicity
COX-2 preferential					
Etodolac	600–1200	7	+	Uncertain	
Meloxicam	7.5–15	24	+	Uncertain	
COX-2 selective					
Celecoxib	200–400	11	+	<1%/year	Not a platelet anticoagulant
Rofecoxib	12.5–25	17	+	<1%/year	Not approved for RA
					Fluid retention with high doses

of about 10:1. Celecoxib and rofecoxib are COX-2 selective; the concentration required to inhibit COX-1 is about 1000 times greater than that required to inhibit COX-2 [13].

The maximum anti-inflammatory potential of the various NSAIDs is approximately equal and is related to the duration of tissue exposure to effective concentrations of drug. For most NSAIDs, gastrointestinal (GI) toxicity associated with COX-1 inhibition limits dosage. This is not the case with selective COX-2 inhibitors; nevertheless, with increasing doses, their efficacy reaches a plateau and further increases in dose do not increase anti-inflammatory benefit. Thus, high doses of aspirin or indomethacin are as effective as the available selective drugs in the suppression of the symptoms of inflammation and fever.

Adverse effects

By far the most important adverse effects of NSAIDs are related to the suppression of COX-1-mediated gastroprotective prostaglandins (which suppress excess gastric acid secretion and help to maintain the gastric mucosal barrier). Loss of gastroprotection results in mucosal hyperemia; diffuse gastritis; and superficial and penetrating ulcers that may be associated with GI bleeding or perforations and sometimes death.

By life table analysis of prospectively collected data from multiple NSAID submissions, the USA Food and Drug Administration (FDA) estimates that GI ulcers, bleeding and perforation occur in approximately 1–2% of patients who use NSAIDs for 3 months and approximately 2–4% of those who use them for 1 year [1]. Based on ARAMIS (Arthritis, Rheumatism and Aging Medical Information System) data, Fries estimated that NSAID-induced gastropathy is responsible for 76,000 hospitalizations and 7600 deaths each year in the United States [14].

Various strategies used to try to improve the gastric tolerability of aspirin and other NSAIDs include: administration with food to dilute the direct gastric irritation; rapidly disintegrating tablets; enteric coated tablets; and timed release dosage forms. Antacids, H_2 blockers and proton pump inhibitors have been used to decrease gastric acid.

Nabumetone is an inactive prodrug in the stomach; after absorption, it is rapidly metabolized to the active NSAID 6-MNA (6-methoxy-2-napthyl acetic acid). 6-MNA is not excreted in the bile and thus has no access to the gastric lumen and causes no direct mucosal irritation. It is therefore an NSAID with better gastric tolerability. It is not used with aspirin or other NSAIDs.

Misoprostil is given with NSAIDs to improve their gastric tolerability. It is an exogenous synthetic prostaglandin analog and is administered orally to replace NSAID-suppressed gastric prostaglandins. Results from a 6-month misoprostil study of 8843 RA patients (mean age 68 years) who continued on NSAIDs revealed that bleeding, perforation or obstruction occurred in 0.5% of patients taking misoprostil (200 µg four times a day) and in 0.95% of patients receiving placebo (P=0.049) [15]. The 0.95% rate of serious upper GI events during 6 months of NSAID treatment in the control group confirms the earlier 2–4% per year estimates of the FDA.

Various advantages and disadvantages of COX-1 and COX-2 inhibition are outlined in Table 4.

Displacement of traditional non-selective COX-1/COX-2 inhibitors has important public health implications and should markedly reduce hospitalizations and deaths caused by the symptomatic treatment of RA.

The role of NSAIDs within the potential management of rheumatoid arthritis

The efficacy of NSAIDs and DMARDs should not be compared. Effective doses of an NSAID relieve many of the symptoms of inflammation without much effect on the underlying progression of the disease. An effective DMARD may completely suppress the disease progression, inducing a remission in some patients. Yet if a physician mistakenly

---

Table 4. Advantages and disadvantages of COX-1 and COX-2 inhibition.

COX-1 inhibition

Advantages

- COX-1 inhibition required for platelet anticoagulation in the treatment of myocardial infarction and strokes

Disadvantages

- Induces potentially lethal gastrointestinal complications

- Associated with decreased glomerular filtration rate and renal failure, especially in patients with marginal renal blood flow that is being supported by renal prostaglandins

- Persistent abnormal transaminase values occurred in 5.4% of RA patients treated with aspirin

COX-2 inhibition

Advantages

- Specific COX-2 inhibition appears markedly to decrease the serious and potentially lethal GI complications of NSAID therapy (in a review of prospective double-blind controlled clinical trials with selective COX-2 inhibitors, the incidence of endoscopically determined gastric erosions or ulcers was similar to that with placebo and much less than that with naproxen or ibuprofen [12])

Disadvantages

- Seems only marginally to improve GI tolerability (in the review of prospective double-blind NSAID-controlled clinical trials with selective COX-2 inhibitors there was no significant reduction in nausea, dyspepsia or abdominal pain [12])

- Specific COX-2 inhibitors cannot replace low-dose aspirin prophylaxis for myocardial infarction or strokes

- Potential adverse effects in brain or reproductive functions; however, they are unlikely to be more severe with specific COX-2 inhibitors than they have been with standard NSAIDs, which also inhibit COX-2

- High doses of the specific COX-2 inhibitor rofecoxib have been associated with edema and a transient decrease in urinary sodium excretion [12]

---

stops an NSAID as soon as a slowly acting DMARD is started, the patient almost immediately notes increased pain, stiffness, swelling and dysfunction, which is relieved by resumption of the NSAID. Corticosteroid efficacy overlaps and surpasses that of NSAIDs. If one is willing to accept the adverse effect liability of corticosteroids, RA patients can be, and frequently are, treated without NSAIDs.

Corticosteroids

Therapeutic administration of corticosteroids produces rapid, potent and reliable suppression of inflammation. Their unsurpassed short-term efficacy and versatility have made corticosteroids a key element in the treatment of many rheumatic diseases (see Table 5) and it is found that in most clinical trials 50% of patients are receiving them.

Interestingly, a decrease in joint erosion progression has been noted in placebo-controlled, prospective studies on patients receiving low-dose daily prednisolone [16]. However, this evidence remains controversial [17].

Various effects of the corticosteroids

Corticosteroids have many effects, including:

1. short-term interference with inflammatory and immune cascades at multiple levels [1]
2. decreasing collagen synthesis and impairing wound healing
3. augmenting gluconeogenesis and glycogen deposition, while inhibiting the action of insulin
4. impairing lipogenesis and stimulating lipolysis in adipose tissue
5. increasing liver synthesis of protein while enhancing its peripheral catabolism
6. interference with intestinal absorption of calcium, inhibiting osteoblast collagen synthesis, elevating parathyroid hormone levels resulting in amplification of osteoclast bone resorption and enhancing renal calcium excretion [18]
7. decreasing immunoglobulin generation, inhibiting immune clearance of sensitized erythrocytes and impairing the transit of immune complexes across basement membranes [18]

Dosage and administration schedule

In general, increasing doses and dosing frequencies of

Table 5. Corticosteroids used in rheumatoid arthritis.

Drug	Relative anti-inflammatory potency	Sodium-retaining potency	Equivalent dose (mg)	Biologic half-life (hours)
Hydrocortisone	1	2+	20	8–12
Prednisone	4	1+	5	12–36
Prednisolone	5	1+	4	12–36
Methylprednisolone	5	0	4	12–36
Triamcinolone	5	0	4	12–36

corticosteroids enhances inflammatory suppression, speeds the onset of therapeutic benefits and increases side effects. For RA, 5–15 mg/day is often used for long periods.

To avoid disease flares after prolonged usage, staged dose reduction is practiced. The reduction is of the order of 0.5–1.0 mg/day every few weeks to months, but should not be more frequent than the time required to detect a steroid dose-related exacerbation of disease activity. In the case of doses below 7 mg/day, the reduction interval must be long enough to allow incremental recovery of adrenal function and this interval will increase with the duration of corticosteroid therapy. Alternate day administration is of limited usefulness in RA because symptoms usually exacerbate during the day without steroids.

For rapid amelioration of damaging inflammation, a short course or even a single large dose can be used. For example, pulsed methylprednisolone, 100–1000 mg/day intravenously for 1–3 days has proven efficacy in the treatment of RA. This may result in profound effects on lymphocyte function leading to a prolonged effect on disease activity, with symptom relief for about 3–6 weeks. However, there is no evidence that it changes the underlying course of the disease [18].

Table 6. Various adverse effects of corticosteroids.

- Increase mortality, shown by Pincus et al. (the data from Fries supported this and indicated that it was not merely a reflection of increased disease severity in those receiving steroids) [19]

- Increase risk of bacterial and opportunistic infections such as tuberculosis, *Pneumocystis carinii* and fungi due to their inhibitory effect on inflammatory and immune responses

- Affect glucose and protein metabolism which may cause hyperglycemia; centripetal fat deposition, leading to rounded facies and a cervical fat pad; and hyperlipidemia

- Cutaneous problems include: capillary fragility, petechiae and easy bruising, acne, hirsutism, impaired wound healing, hyperhidrosis and striae

- Glaucoma and cataract formation

- Further complications include: hypokalemia, fluid retention, edema, hypertension, myopathy, possible ulcerogenicity, pancreatitis, premature atherosclerosis, avascular necrosis of bone, psychiatric disturbances and bowel or diverticular perforations

---

Adverse effects

The adverse effects of corticosteroid usage are summarized in Table 6.

High-dose steroids can mask the symptoms of infections or other inflammatory processes, making diagnosis difficult. One-gram pulses may induce cardiac arrhythmia in hypokalemic patients and may result in the hematogenous dissemination of previously localized infections. Concomitant illnesses or previous adverse reactions may guide the physician when prescribing corticosteroids.

Disease-modifying anti-rheumatic drugs

The term 'disease-modifying anti-rheumatic drug' (DMARD) refers to a group of medications with diverse mechanisms of action that have traditionally been used if RA is not improving with NSAIDs and other conservative treatment modalities. Examples include: gold compounds, chloroquine, hydroxychloroquine, sulfasalazine, D-penicillamine, azathioprine and methotrexate, as well as cyclosporine A, minocycline, leflunomide and tumor necrosis factor (TNF) inhibitors such as etanercept and infliximab (see Table 7). They produce additional clinical benefit when added to continuing stable background NSAID and low-dose corticosteroid therapy. Although a few long-term responders continue treatment with gold compounds, D-penicillamine and azathioprine, their use has markedly diminished in the past 10 years, because their relatively poor risk to benefit ratios lead to frequent discontinuation for toxicity or loss of benefit.

DMARDs differ from NSAIDs by their usually delayed onset of action and lack of analgesia. They appear to act more proximally on the inflammatory process, perhaps on the immunologic initiators of tissue injury, but without removing the basic cause of RA. It generally takes weeks or months of treatment before clinical benefit is recognized and this is perhaps because their proximal effects take considerable time to influence the intermediate and distal sites of inflammation. However, TNF inhibition may produce benefit within 24–48 hours in some patients.

Important properties of DMARDs are as follows:

1. DMARDs most often only moderate the disease process and some level of chronic inflammation generally persists
2. if a drug-induced remission does occur, it is likely that the disease will recur within weeks to months after the drug is discontinued
3. the disease may exacerbate even when the drug is being maintained at the same dose (this phenomenon is not well understood)
4. DMARDs often decrease acute phase reactants and may slow the rate of progression of joint damage and disability [1,7,9]

Table 7. DMARDs in the year 2000 (excluding biologicals).

Drug	Dose	TOXICITY Efficacy	Treatment limiting	Potentially severe	Suggested monitoring
Methotrexate	5.0–25 mg PO or IM once weekly	+++	++	Hepatic fibrosis, acute interstitial pneumonitis, bone marrow suppression	Baseline chest radiograph and hepatitis B, C serologies
					CBC every 2–4 weeks for 4 months, then every 4 weeks
					Liver function tests every 4–8 weeks
					Creatinine levels every 4–8 weeks
Sulfasalazine	500–3000 mg/day PO	+++	++	Bone marrow suppression	Baseline G6PD
					CBC every 2 weeks for 8 weeks, then monthly for 6 months, then every 2–3 months
					Liver function tests every 2–3 months
Hydroxychloro-quine sulfate	400 mg/day PO	++	+	Rare retinal toxicity	Ophthalmologic examination (baseline, then every 6 months)
Cyclosporine	2.5–4 mg/kg/day PO	++*	++	Renal dysfunction, hypertension	Creatinine every 2 weeks for 3 months, then monthly
					Decrease dose if creatinine increases ≥25% above baseline
Leflunomide	Loading dose: 100 mg/day x 3 days Maintenance: 20 mg/day	+++	++	New drug, uncertain	Same as methotrexate

Adapted from Borigini MJ, Paulus HE. Rheumatoid arthritis. In: Weisman MH, Weinblatt ME, Louie J, editors. Treatment of Rheumatoid Arthritis 2nd ed. Philadelphia: WB Saunders, 2000.
CBC: complete blood count; G6PD: glucose-6-phosphate dehydrogenase; PO: by mouth; IM: intramuscular.
Efficacy and toxicity estimates based on [54,55].
*Efficacy increased when used with methotrexate

Methotrexate

RA was first treated with an antifolate by Gubner in 1951, but it was not until the 1980s that methotrexate became an acceptable option in the treatment of RA. During the 1990s it has become the DMARD of choice for most RA patients [1,20] and it is currently the most commonly used DMARD for RA.

Mechanism of action

Methotrexate and its polyglutamates are direct inhibitors of thymidylate synthase and folate dependent enzymes of purine biosynthesis, such as dihydrofolate reductase. Such blockades may alter purine biosynthesis, producing immunosuppression by secondary inhibition of crucial enzymes and perhaps also by decreasing leukotriene B_4 production, interleukin-1 and -6 expression and phospholipase A_2 activity [20,22].

Dosage/Efficacy

Methotrexate has a significant anti-inflammatory effect within 3–8 weeks after starting therapy; it is usually taken one day a week in doses of 5–25 mg, depending on efficacy and toxic reactions, and has remained effective for as long as 84 months of treatment [20]. The once weekly dosing schedule was arrived at by trial and error and is crucially important to minimize toxicity whilst still retaining acceptable efficacy in RA. Inhibition of dihydrofolate reductase is incomplete during weekly low-dose methotrexate and may not be essential for efficacy [21].

Clinical trials/Observational studies

Randomized, placebo-controlled clinical trials in the 1980s demonstrated short-term clinical benefits [23,24] and long-term efficacy [25,26]. After 5 years, 50% of methotrexate-treated RA patients were still receiving methotrexate, as compared to 15–20% for other DMARDs such as gold salts or D-penicillamine [26].

Long-term observational studies with the use of methotrexate in RA patients have demonstrated an acceptable toxicity profile as well as sustained clinical benefit and decreased radiographic progression of joint damage. Recent data suggest that methotrexate therapy may improve life expectancy even in patients with advanced RA [27].

The recently published placebo-controlled trial comparing methotrexate to leflunomide demonstrated that both of these drugs were superior to placebo in slowing radiographic progression of disease [7].

Adverse effects

Toxicity is the major factor limiting the clinical usefulness of methotrexate [26]. Methotrexate is cleared, to a certain extent, through the kidneys. Therefore the dosage must be decreased in patients with mild renal insufficiency and it should not be used in patients with renal failure or on dialysis. In methotrexate patients, leukopenia and thrombocytopenia have rarely been associated with an NSAID-induced decrease in glomerular filtration and inhibition of renal tubular secretion [20].

GI manifestations (stomatitis, nausea, vomiting and/or diarrhea) have been reported to occur in as many as 60% of methotrexate-treated RA patients [20]. Many GI manifestations can be alleviated by the concomitant administration of folic acid, or a change in route of administration (from oral to parenteral) [21]. Toxicity may be further diminished by folinic acid (leukovorin), 5 mg, 8–12 hours after the weekly dose of methotrexate, thus bypassing the dihydrofolate reductase block [20].

The occurrence of liver damage after prolonged administration of methotrexate for RA was a matter of serious concern in the 1980s based on previous experience with the drug in the treatment of psoriasis [28]. It has now become evident that clinically significant liver disease is less frequent than previously predicted. Risk factors for methotrexate-induced hepatic cirrhosis include: long duration of treatment with methotrexate, advancing age and ethanol abuse. The potential toxicities of methotrexate in the treatment of RA patients have resulted in the American College of Rheumatology (ACR) developing guidelines to monitor for some of these events [29].

Although uncommon, an acute pulmonary syndrome/allergic pneumonitis (cough, progressive dyspnea and markedly decreased oxygenation) is a potentially severe, and an occasionally fatal, adverse event; this usually improves with prompt discontinuance of the drug [30]. Infectious processes need to be ruled out in this clinical setting.

Further complications that may occur include reversible bone marrow suppression, occasional systemic fungal infections and other unusual infections [20]. Methotrexate is contraindicated in pregnancy because of a high probability of teratogenesis.

Sulfasalazine

Many physicians use the weaker antifolate, sulfasalazine, for patients with mild RA; it is one of the few DMARDs specifically developed to treat RA [31]. Sulfasalazine is a chemical combination of a salicylate and a sulfa moiety and is contraindicated in patients with sulfa or salicylate allergies.

Mechanism of action

It has been postulated that its mechanism of action may be similar to that of methotrexate; however, it remains undefined.

Dosage/Efficacy

The usual starting dose is 500 or 1000 mg/day, slowly raised to 2 or 3 g/day over a 4–6 week period, an approach which may decrease adverse reactions [31]. The rate of continuation of sulfasalazine is comparable to that of other DMARDs, i.e. 22% at 5 years.

Clinical trials/Observational studies

Reports from McConkey et al. suggested beneficial effects with sulfasalazine in RA [32]. Several controlled clinical trials have also indicated efficacy in RA [31,33]. Sulfasalazine decreases the progression rate of radiographic joint erosions, compared to placebo [7].

Adverse effects

Approximately 30% of patients discontinue sulfasalazine because of adverse events, which are usually benign and reversible with drug discontinuation. Dose-related and acetylator-phenotype dependent effects include nausea, vomiting, headache, malaise, hemolytic anemia, reticulocytosis and methemoglobinemia [33]. Other adverse events appear to be hypersensitivity reactions and include rashes, aplastic anemia and autoimmune hemolysis.

Antimalarials (hydroxychloroquine and chloroquine)

Early controlled trials of the antimalarials: chloroquine and hydroxychloroquine, showed suppression of rheumatoid joint inflammation [34]. Hydroxychloroquine is the least toxic DMARD. Most clinicians would agree that the place of hydroxychloroquine in the sequence of DMARD use is in early mild disease and they often continue it as a background therapy when another DMARD is started. Controlled, multicenter studies on early RA show decreased joint inflammation and stiffness with few significant side effects [35,36]. Antimalarial drugs are also effective in juvenile rheumatoid arthritis (JRA) [36].

Mechanism of action

The antimalarial compounds are weak bases. At the neutral pH of serum, they diffuse into acidic vacuoles where they become protonated. The more polar protonated molecules are unable to diffuse out of the vacuoles and so the pH within the vacuole increases by 1–2 pH units, which alters the molecular assembly of α-β-peptide complexes. This may interfere with antigenic processing, reduce stimulation of autoimmune CD4+ T cells and down-regulate autoimmune responses [37]. Antimalarials can interfere with the 'presentation of antigen' to T cells by macrophages [36]. Chloroquine has been shown to decrease antigen processing and presentation by both macrophages and lymphoid dendritic cells [36].

Additional proposed mechanisms of action include the following: inhibition of DNA polymerase; interference with phospholipase A_1; interference with neutrophil superoxide release; and inhibition of cytokine release, including interleukin-1 (IL-1), TNF and interferon-γ [36]. These mechanisms would be expected to result in a rapid onset of anti-inflammatory activity (similar to corticosteroids or NSAIDs); however, the clinical onset of benefit after starting antimalarial drugs takes several months.

Dosage/Efficacy

Hydroxychloroquine's onset of action is delayed: response is seen in 40–60% of patients by 3–6 months, but it may take 9–12 months for maximum response to occur [34]. As a quinolone, it is well-absorbed and extensively distributed, with high concentrations in liver, lung, kidney, heart and pigmented tissues. Excretion is slow and may continue for as long as 5 years after the drug is discontinued.

Hydroxychloroquine's initial efficacy and lack of reported toxicity during the 1950–1960 period led to escalation of daily doses up to 10–15 mg/kg/day. Ocular toxicity with hydroxychloroquine was first reported in 1967 [34]. From 1960–1989, 18 cases of retinopathy in patients receiving hydroxychloroquine were reported either in the literature or to the FDA; in 16 of these cases, the dose of hydroxychloroquine was greater than 7 mg/kg/day [38]. A recent review of the ophthalmology literature supports the safety of hydroxychloroquine at a dose of 6–7 mg/kg/day in patients without renal failure, i.e. about 400 mg/day in an average weight woman [38].

Clinical trials/Observational studies

To investigate whether dose-loading of hydroxychloroquine increases benefit in treating RA, a study was performed where RA patients with mild disease were randomized to receive either 400, 800 or 1200 mg/day for 6 weeks, followed by 400 mg/day [40]. The degree of initial clinical response was increased in those patients who received the highest doses. Short-term ocular toxicity was not dose-related but GI toxicity was.

Adverse effects

Retinal toxicity has been reported in patients receiving hydroxychloroquine. The high concentrations found in the pigment layers of the retina may lead to retinal damage with destruction of rods and cones. Significant retinopathy is very rare with current dosing regimens [38]. Early changes can be detected by an electro-retinogram or by changes in color vision or visual fields; in a patient without symptoms, abnormal results in a sensitive ophthalmologic examination occur in 0.5–10% of patients. If clinical symptoms of visual impairment occur, the damage may be irreversible. Therefore, patients undergo an ophthalmologic examination for retinopathy before starting hydroxychloroquine and periodically thereafter [38]. The drug should be stopped at the first sign of retinal toxicity. The issue of cumulative-dose toxicity with hydroxychloroquine remains controversial, but several reports indicate the risks are low [39]. Other side effects include dermatitis, nausea and epigastric pain, insomnia, myopathy, headache, hemolytic anemia and rare leukopenia. All side effects, however, are extremely infrequent.

Cyclosporine

Cyclosporine is a standard immunosuppressive drug for the prevention of organ rejection in heart, liver and kidney transplants.

Mechanism of action

It has variable antifungal properties; it complexes with cytoplasmic-binding proteins, called immunophilins, which appear to be essential for the immunosuppressive effects. It produces specific reversible inhibition of T-lymphocytes and inhibition of lymphokine production and release.

Dosage/Efficacy

Doses of 2.5–4.0 mg/kg/day in RA patients are more effective than placebo [41]. However, it is usually used in combination with methotrexate. Clinical responses after 6 months' treatment with the combination were markedly better than those in patients who continued methotrexate (plus placebo) and were better than those with cyclosporine alone [42]. This suggested a beneficial interaction between cyclosporine and methotrexate [43].

Adverse effects

Serum creatinine must be monitored frequently in patients treated with cyclosporine, because it causes dose-related impairment of renal function and hypertension, usually with doses greater than 5 mg/kg/day. A 25% or greater increase above pre-treatment creatinine levels mandates a decrease in dosage, which is usually associated with a decrease in creatinine. Persistent dosing despite rising creatinine values may cause an irreversible decrease of renal function.

Leflunomide

Leflunomide was approved in 1998 for the treatment of RA.

Mechanism of action

Leflunomide is a prodrug that is slowly absorbed; its active metabolite inhibits dihydroorotate dehydrogenase, thus inhibiting pyrimidine biosynthesis [44].

Dosage/Efficacy

It is slowly excreted in urine and stool with a long half-life of about 16 days, taking about 7–8 weeks to reach steady-state levels in the blood. In order to decrease the time to reach steady-state, a loading dose of 100 mg/day for 3 days is recommended, followed by maintenance doses of 20 mg/day. Cholestyramine can be given to enhance fecal elimination, decreasing the half-life to about 24 hours. Leflunomide is highly protein-bound and may increase concentrations of diclofenac, ibuprofen and tolbutamide, but not of warfarin or methotrexate. Rifampin increases leflunomide concentrations by about 40%.

Clinical trials/Observational studies

In clinical trials, leflunomide efficacy was similar to that of methotrexate and sulfasalazine. The onset of benefit is relatively rapid, with significant benefit after 1–3 months of treatment [45,46]. The rate of progression of radiographic damage to hand/wrist and forefoot joints during a 12 month study was significantly less than that with placebo and comparable to that with methotrexate [7].

Adverse effects

Leflunomide use is not recommended in patients with significant hepatic impairment or with positive hepatitis B or C serologies. Abnormal liver function tests (ALT or AST) occurred in about 30% of patients on leflunomide, compared to 11% on placebo. Most abnormalities reversed during continued treatment, or lowering the dose to 10 mg/day, but liver function tests should be monitored monthly initially and patients with levels ≥3 times normal should be discontinued. Leflunomide is teratogenic and is contraindicated during pregnancy. It may take up to 2 years after discontinuation to completely excrete leflunomide and so pregnancy should be avoided until plasma levels are less than 0.03 mg/l. This may be achieved more quickly by giving cholestyramine 8 g three times a day for 10 days [1].

Minocycline

In the late 1960s, several reports described improvement in patients with RA after treatment with tetracycline. Minocycline has been studied in patients with RA. Its role in clinical practice is uncertain. Although some improvement was noted for the patients on minocycline in a study undertaken by the National Institutes of Health, placebo response was also high [47]. In a Dutch study, patients with a long history of disease derived significant benefit from treatment with minocycline compared with placebo [48]. Vertigo was a drug-related side effect and was associated with falls and fractures in two patients.

DMARD combination therapy

Although methotrexate is continued for over 5 years by more than 50% of patients, few patients with RA are in complete remission and many, if not most, may be candidates for the addition of another DMARD [25,26]. The use of combinations of DMARDs when a single DMARD fails adequately to control RA is now generally accepted by rheumatologists.

A 1997 survey of 200 USA rheumatologists found that combination DMARD therapy was used by 99% of rheumatologists to treat an estimated 24% of their RA patients [49]. Methotrexate with hydroxychloroquine was the most frequently used combination. In 1990, a review of DMARD combination studies reported that early anecdotal reports and uncontrolled trials found various DMARD combinations to be effective; however, *de novo* balanced, randomized prospective clinical trials showed no advantage to combinations when compared with each of their component single DMARDs [50]. Three observations of DMARD combination therapy are outlined below:

1. a prospective randomized study (published in 1997) of either methotrexate, sulfasalazine or the combination as the first DMARD therapy in 115 early RA patients showed no significant differences between the three treatment groups after 1 year, although there was a trend toward greater improvement with the combination [51]

2. triple DMARD therapy with methotrexate, sulfasalazine and hydroxychloroquine was more effective than methotrexate alone or a sulfasalazine/hydroxychloroquine combination in patients who had experienced a poor response to single DMARD therapy with one or more of the three DMARDs, or gold or penicillamine [52]

3. the COBRA trial in 155 patients with only 4 months of RA demonstrated that a step-down combination of high dose prednisolone (60 mg/day tapering to 7.5 mg after 6 weeks and 0 mg after 35 weeks), methotrexate (7.5 mg/week for 46 weeks) and sulfasalazine (2 g/day) was more effective than sulfasalazine alone until the prednisolone was stopped. After the prednisolone was stopped, the clinical differences between the treatment arms were no longer significant, but radiographic joint damage was less in the combined therapy group [53]

Methotrexate is the most commonly used 'anchor drug' in combination therapy. Evidence from randomized, placebo-controlled clinical trials has indicated increased efficacy and acceptable (and often lower) toxicity in patients who have tolerated, but had inadequate benefit with, methotrexate when cyclosporine, sulfasalazine, etanercept or infliximab is added. Further studies and long-term follow-up are needed to determine the long-term effectiveness, toxicities and optimal clinical use of DMARD combinations.

Conclusions

There is general agreement that rheumatoid inflammation should be controlled as completely as possible, as soon as possible and that this control should be maintained for as long as possible, consistent with patient safety. The risk of RA management has decreased as rheumatologists have gained more experience with methotrexate and using combinations of DMARDs, and as increasingly specific and less toxic agents (e.g. TNF inhibitors, COX-2 inhibitors) have become available to modify inflammation. Evidence that a number of interventions can retard the progression of joint damage has increased the potential benefit of therapy. Improved therapeutic risk/benefit and the progressive, irreversible nature of RA joint damage justify immediate initiation of DMARD treatment of newly diagnosed RA and this is rapidly becoming the expected standard of care.

Unfortunately, most patients achieve only partial suppression of rheumatoid inflammation and many lose therapeutic benefit after an initial good response. Additive combination therapy is the usual response to this, but also may produce only temporary benefit. Even in patients with a complete response, RA manifestations almost always recur after the treatment is stopped. The management of persistent or recurrent rheumatoid inflammation and disability continues to be a challenge.

References

1. Borigini MJ, Paulus HE. Rheumatoid arthritis. In: Weisman MH, Weinblatt ME, Louie J, editors. Treatment of Rheumatoid Arthritis 2nd ed. Philadelphia: WB Saunders, 2000.

2. Scott DL, Symmons DPM, Coulton B et al. Long-term outcome of treating rheumatoid arthritis: results after 20 years. Lancet 1987;1:1108–11.

3. Pincus T, Callahan LF. Taking mortality in rheumatoid arthritis seriously—predictive markers, socioeconomic status and comorbidity. J Rheumatol 1986;13:841–5.

4. van der Heide A, Jacobs JWG, Bijlsma JWJ. The effectiveness of early treatment with 'second-line' antirheumatic drugs: a randomized, controlled trial. Ann Intern Med 1996;124:699–707.

5. Egsmose C, Lund B, Borg C et al. Patients with rheumatoid arthritis benefit from early 2nd line therapy: 5 year follow-up of a prospective double blind placebo controlled study. J Rheumatol 1995;22:2208–13.

6. Ten Wolde S, Breedveld FC, Hermans J et al. Randomised placebo-controlled study of stopping second-line drugs in rheumatoid arthritis. Lancet 1996;347:347–52.

7. Sharp JT, Strand V, Leung H et al. Treatment with leflunomide slows radiographic progression of RA. Results from three randomized controlled trials of leflunomide in patients with active rheumatoid arthritis. Arthritis Rheum 2000;43:495–505.

8. Lipsky PE, van der Heijde DMFM, St Clair EW at al. Infliximab and methotrexate in the treatment of rheumatoid arthritis. N Engl J Med 2000;343:1594–602.

9. Bathon JM, Martin RW, Fleischmann RM et al. A comparison of etanercept and methotrexate in patients with early rheumatoid arthritis. N Engl J Med 2000;343:1586–93.

10. Vane JR. Inhibition of prostaglandin synthesis as the mechanism of action for aspirin-like drugs. Nature New Biol 1971;231:232–5.

11. Masferrer JL, Zweifel BS, Seibert K et al. Selective regulation of cellular cyclooxygenase by dexamethasone and endotoxin in mice. J Clin Invest 1990;86:1375–9.

12. Crofford LJ, Lipsky PE, Brooks P et al. Basic biology and clinical application of specific cyclooxygenase-2 inhibitors. Arthritis Rheum 2000;43:4–13.

13. Furst DE. Pharmacology and efficacy of cyclooxygenase (COX) inhibitors. Am J Med 1999;107(Suppl.):18S–26S.

14. Fries JF. NSAID gastropathy: the second most deadly rheumatic disease? Epidemiology and risk appraisal. J Rheumatol 1991;18(Suppl. 28):6–10.

15. Silverstein FE, Graham DY, Senior JR et al. Misoprostil reduces serious gastrointestinal complications in patients with rheumatoid arthritis receiving nonsteroidal anti-inflammatory drugs. Ann Intern Med 1995;123:241–9.

16. Kirwan JR and the Arthritis & Rheumatism Council Low Dose Glucocorticoid Study Group. The effect of glucocorticoids on joint destruction in rheumatoid arthritis. N England J Med 1995;333:142–6.

17. Paulus HE, Di Primeo D, Sanda M et al. Progression of radiographic joint erosion during low-dose corticosteroid treatment of rheumatoid arthritis. J Rheumatol 2000;27:1632–7.

18. Garber EK, Targoff C, Paulus HE. Corticosteroids in the rheumatic diseases: chronic low doses, chronic high doses, 'pulses', intra-articular. In: Paulus HE, Furst DE, Dromgoole SH, editors. Drugs for Rheumatic Disease. New York: Churchill Livingstone, 1987:443.

19. Pincus T, Marcum SB, Callahan LF. Long term drug therapy for RA in seven rheumatology private practices: 2nd line drugs and prednisone. J Rheumatol 1992;19:1885–94.

20. Weinblatt ME. Methotrexate. In: Kelley WN, Harris ED Jr, Ruddy S, Sledge CB, editors. Textbook of Rheumatology 5th ed Philadelphia: WB Saunders, 1997:771.

21. Morgan SL, Baggott JE, Vaughn WH et al. The effect of folic acid supplementation on the toxicity of low-dose methotrexate treatment in patients with rheumatoid arthritis. Arthritis Rheum 1990;33:9–18.

22. van der Veen MJ, van der Heide A, Kruize AA et al. Infection rate and use of antibiotics in patients with rheumatoid arthritis treated with methotrexate. Ann Rheum Dis 1994;53:224–8.

23. Weinblatt ME, Coblyn JS, Fox DA et al. Efficacy of low-dose methotrexate in rheumatoid arthritis. N Engl J Med 1985;312:818–22.

24. Williams HJ, Wilkens RF, Samuelson CO Jr et al. Comparison of low-dose oral pulse methotrexate and placebo in the treatment of rheumatoid arthritis. A controlled clinical trial. Arthritis Rheum 1985;28:721–30.

25. Buchbinder R, Hall S, Sambrook PN et al. Methotrexate therapy in rheumatoid arthritis: a life table review of 587 patients treated in community practice. J Rheumatol 1993;20:639–44.

26. Alarcon GS, Trace IC, Blackburn WD Jr. Methotrexate in rheumatoid arthritis. Toxic effects as the major factor in limiting long-term treatment. Arthritis Rheum 1989;32:671–6.

27. Krause D, Schleusser B, Herborn G et al. Response to methotrexate treatment is associated with reduced mortality in patients with severe rheumatoid arthritis. Arthritis Rheum 2000;43:14–21.

28. Kremer JM, Galivan J, Streckfuss A et al. Methotrexate metabolism analysis in blood and liver of rheumatoid arthritis patients. Association with hepatic folate deficiency and formation of polyglutamates. Arthritis Rheum 1986;29:832–5.

29. Kremer JM, Alarcon GS, Lightfoot RW Jr et al. Methotrexate for rheumatoid arthritis. Suggested guidelines for monitoring liver toxicity. Arthritis Rheum 1994;37:316–28.

30. Alarcon GS, Gispen JG, Koopman WJ. Severe reversible interstitial pneumonitis induced by low dose methotrexate. J Rheumatol 1989;16:1007–8.

31. Day RO. Sulfasalazine. In: Kelley WN, Harris ED Jr, Ruddy S, Sledge CB, editors. Textbook of Rheumatology 5th ed. Philadelphia: WB Saunders, 1997:741.

32. McConkey B, Amos RS, Durham S et al. Sulphasalazine in rheumatoid arthritis. Br Med J 1980;280:442–4.

33. Williams HJ, Ward JR, Dahl SL et al. A controlled trial comparing sulfasalazine, gold sodium thiomalate and placebo in rheumatoid arthritis. Arthritis Rheum 1988;31:702–13.

34. Wickens S, Paulus HE. Antimalarial drugs. In: Paulus HE, Furst DE, Dromgoole SH, editors. Drugs for Rheumatic Disease. New York: Churchill Livingstone, 1987:113.

35. HERA. A randomized trial of hydroxychloroquine in early rheumatoid arthritis: the HERA study. Am J Med 1995;98:156–68.

36. Rynes RI. Antimalarial drugs. In: Kelley WN, Harris ED Jr, Ruddy S. Sledge CB, editors. Textbook of Rheumatology 5th ed. Philadelphia: WB Saunders, 1997:747.

37. Fox RI, Kang H. Mechanism of action of antimalarial drugs: inhibition of antigen processing and presentation. Lupus 1993;2(Suppl. 1):S9–12.

38. Bernstein HN. Ocular safety of hydroxychloroquine. Ann Ophthalmol 1991;23:292–6.

39. Rynes R. Ophthalmologic safety of long-term hydroxychloroquine sulfate treatment. Am J Med 1983;75:35–9.

40. Furst DE, Lindsley H, Baethage B et al. Dose-loading with hydroxychloroquine improves the rate of response in early, active rheumatoid arthritis. Arthritis Rheum 1999;42:357–65.

41. Tugwell P, Bombardier C, Gent M et al. Low-dose cyclosporin versus placebo in patients with rheumatoid arthritis. Lancet 1990;335:1051–5.

42. Tugwell P, Pincus T, Yocum D et al. Combination therapy with cyclosporine and methotrexate in severe rheumatoid arthritis. N Engl J Med 1995;333:137–41.

43. Fox R, Morgan S, Smith H et al. Treatment of RA patients with methotrexate plus cyclosporine A leads to elevation of plasma methotrexate levels and decrease of hydroxy-methotrexate levels. Arthritis Rheum 1998;41(Suppl. 9):S138.

44. Fox R, Mahboubi A, Green D et al. Leflunomide inhibits de novo uridine synthesis and is dependent on p53 for arrest in G1 phase of cell cycle. Arthritis Rheum 1998; 41(Suppl. 9):S137.

45. Mladenovic V, Domljan Z, Rozman B et al. Safety and effectiveness of leflunomide in the treatment of patients with active rheumatoid arthritis. Arthritis Rheum 1995;38:1595–603.

46. Weaver A, Caldwell J, Olsen H et al. Treatment of active rheumatoid arthritis with leflunomide compared to methotrexate. Arthritis Rheum 1998;41(Suppl. 9):S131.

47. Tilley BC, Alarcón GS, Heyse SP et al. Minocycline in rheumatoid arthritis. A 48-week, double-blind, placebo-controlled trial. MIRA Trial Group. Ann Intern Med 1995;122:81–9.

48. Kloppenburg M, Breedveld FC, Terwiel JP et al. Minocycline in active rheumatoid arthritis. A double-blind, placebo-controlled trial. Arthritis Rheum 1994;37:629–36.

49. O'Dell J. Combination DMARD therapy for rheumatoid arthritis: apparent universal acceptance. Arthritis Rheum 1997;40(Suppl.):50.

50. Paulus HE. Current controversies in rheumatology: The use of combinations of disease-modifying anti-rheumatic agents in rheumatoid arthritis. Arthritis Rheum 1990;33:113–20.

51. Haagsma CJ, van Riel PLCM, de Jong AJL et al. Combination of sulfasalazine and methotrexate versus the single components in early rheumatoid arthritis: a randomized, controlled, double-blind 52 week clinical trial. Br J Rheumatol 1997;36:1082–8.

52. O'Dell JR, Haire CE, Erikson N et al. Treatment of rheumatoid arthritis with methotrexate alone, sulfasalazine and hydroxychloroquine or a combination of all three medications. N Engl J Med 1996;334:1287–91.

53. Boers M, Verhoeven AC, Markusse HM et al. Randomized comparison of combined step-down prednisolone, methotrexate and sulfasalazine with sulfasalazine alone in early rheumatoid arthritis. Lancet 1997;350:309–18.

54. Felson DT, Anderson JJ, Meenan RF. The comparative efficacy and toxicity of second-line drugs in rheumatoid arthritis. Arthritis Rheum 1990;33(10):1449-61.

55. Felson DT, Anderson JJ, Meenan RF. Use of short-term efficacy/toxicity tradeoffs to select second-line agents in rheumatoid arthritis. Arthritis Rheum 1992;35(10):1117-25.

5

Cytokine therapies: targeting tumor necrosis factor and interleukin -1

Arthur Kavanaugh

Over the past few decades, the immunopathogenesis of rheumatoid arthritis (RA) has become increasingly well delineated. Research from numerous laboratories has helped unravel the dysregulation of immunocompetent cells and their secreted products that is characteristic of RA. Accompanying this progress and in concert with advances in biopharmaceutical development, there has been a growing expectation that novel immunomodulatory agents might emerge that would expand the therapeutic approach to this debilitating condition. Recently, biologic response modifiers have been introduced that inhibit the function of the key pro-inflammatory cytokines: tumor necrosis factor-α (TNF-α) and interleukin-1 (IL-1). These agents have shown considerable efficacy in research trials as well as substantial effectiveness in early clinical experience.

Immunopathogenesis of rheumatoid arthritis

RA is a chronic, progressive disease of unknown etiology. The initiation of this aggressive systemic inflammatory disorder presumably results from exposure of a genetically susceptible host to some as yet unidentified environmental stimulus [1,2]. The propagation and sustenance of inflammation reflect an active and ongoing, immunologically driven process. Several components of the immune response are intimately involved in the pathogenesis of RA. Changes in the vasculature occur early in the disease course and facilitate its propagation. Such changes include angiogenesis and alteration of the endothelium into an activated, 'high endothelial venule' phenotype.

Re-circulating CD4+ T lymphocytes, particularly those with a memory phenotype, accrue in the synovium utilizing specific adhesion molecules. These T cells, many of which have a Th1 pattern of cytokine secretion, play a central role in the initiation and orchestration of the autoimmune response.

Resident synovial cells such as fibroblasts, macrophages, dendritic cells, mast cells, endothelial cells as well as blood-derived B cells are crucial contributors to rheumatoid inflammation [1-3]. Interactions among these various cells result in the liberation of various mediators, such as cytokines, prostaglandins and many others. These soluble mediators produce local tissue damage and cause many of the signs and symptoms of disease. In addition, some mediators, particularly cytokines, exert prominent stimulatory effects on cells, thereby propagating the chronic yet dynamic immunologic response underlying rheumatoid inflammation.

Cytokines are small peptide molecules typically released from cells upon activation. By binding specific cell surface receptors, they can exert a myriad of biologic functions; cytokines may exhibit pleiotropy (i.e. one cytokine can mediate diverse functions), redundancy (i.e. several cytokines may mediate the same activity) or antagonism (i.e. the effects of one cytokine may be inhibited by another cytokine or by soluble forms of the cytokine receptor) [4,5]. While cytokines can be considered individually, *in vivo* they function in complex networks and cascades. Thus the overall outcome of a response reflects the balance between pro-inflammatory factors (e.g. inflammatory cytokines) and anti-inflammatory factors (e.g. soluble forms of cytokine receptors and cytokines with anti-inflammatory function) present in the local milieu.

In RA, there is substantial evidence that cytokines, particularly pro-inflammatory cytokines such as TNF-α and IL-1, subserve a crucial role in disease expression and propagation [1-5]. Thus, these cytokines may be particularly appropriate therapeutic targets in RA [6,7]. A number of recent trials have used varied methods to modulate the availability or function of these key mediators.

Cytokines: tumor necrosis factor (TNF) and interleukin-1 (IL-1)

Tumor necrosis factor

TNF, the prototype of a family of molecules involved in immune regulation and inflammation, was named for its ability to induce necrosis of tumors when injected into certain tumor-bearing animals. Although the initial observation of this effect was made in the 1890s, most knowledge of the role of TNF has been ascertained over the past 2 decades [8]. Soon after it was cloned in 1984, TNF was found to be identical to another molecule that had been called 'cachectin'; it was also found to be approximately 30% homologous to the molecule known as 'lymphotoxin' (LT). Genes encoding both TNF-α and the two forms of LT (LT-α and LT-β) are closely linked on chromosome 6, between loci for Class I and Class II molecules of the major histocompatibility complex (MHC).

Although it can be synthesized and secreted by various types of cells, at inflammatory sites TNF-α is produced primarily by macrophages in response to various pro-inflammatory stimuli such as bacterial lipopolysaccharide. Production of TNF-α is closely regulated at transcriptional and post-transcriptional levels (e.g. mRNA stability and translational efficiency). TNF-α is synthesized and expressed as a 26 kD transmembrane protein and can be functional on the cell surface. However, as a result of proteolytic cleavage by a specific metalloproteinase (referred to as TNF-α converting enzyme, or TACE), it is cleaved and released from the cell surface. Secreted TNF-α functions as a soluble homotrimer of 17 kD subunits. LT-α, which was previously called TNF-β, also functions as a soluble homotrimer; it is produced and secreted almost exclusively by lymphocytes after antigenic or mitogenic stimulation.

Both TNF-α and LT-α bind to two specific cell surface receptors: the 55 kD (also referred to as CD120a or TNF-RI) and the 75 kD (also referred to as CD120b or TNF-RII) TNF receptors [8]. These receptors, which are type I transmembrane proteins, are present on numerous cell types. It is thought that CD120a and CD120b can mediate overlapping activities in most tissues, although potentially important differences between the receptors have been noted in affinity for ligand, signaling properties and some aspects of function [8–10]. Soluble forms of both CD120a and CD120b, which bind TNF-α or LT-α with high avidity and compete with cell surface receptors for binding, can be detected in blood, where they may serve an inhibitory function. Elevated concentrations of these receptors can be demonstrated in the synovial fluid of patients with RA. LT-β, which functions as a heterotrimer of one LT-α and two LT-β subunits, is a transmembrane protein present on the surface of T cells and some other cells. LT-β does not bind to the 55 kD or 75 kD TNF-Rs; rather, it binds to a distinct cell surface receptor (LT-βR).

TNF and the TNF receptors are members of families of related pairs of co-receptor molecules that include: Fas-ligand (FasL)/Fas (CD95), CD40L (CD154)/CD40, CD27L (CD70)/CD27, CD30L/CD30 and others. Signaling cascades initiated by these receptor/counter-receptor interactions include activation of transcription factors (e.g. nuclear factor-kappa B [NF-κB]), protein kinases (e.g. MAPK, JNK, p38) and proteases (e.g. caspases). Molecules in this family can play key roles not only in the activation of cells, but also in programmed cell death (i.e. apoptosis).

Interleukin-1

There are three members of the IL-1 gene family: IL-1α, IL-1β and IL-1 receptor antagonist (IL-1Ra), and two IL-1 receptors (IL-1RI, IL-1RII); all are encoded on chromosome 2 [7,11,12]. IL-1α is synthesized as a 31 kD precursor that acts largely within cells, probably as an autocrine growth factor. However, IL-1α can be expressed and can function on the cell surface. IL-1β is synthesized as pro-IL-1β, which is not fully active within the cytosol. After cleavage by the IL-1β converting enzyme (ICE; also known as caspase 1), 17 kD IL-1β is secreted and is fully functional. IL-1 is synthesized in response to numerous stimuli. Although a variety of cells can secrete IL-1, at inflammatory sites such as the rheumatoid synovium macrophages are the most important source.

The IL-1 system is unique among cytokines because of the endogenous inhibitor, IL-1Ra. There are several forms of IL-1Ra. One is secreted, and functions as a competitive inhibitor of IL-1α and IL-1β by binding to the same counter-receptor but transducing no signal. Other forms of IL-1Ra are intracellular; although they may also serve inhibitory functions, their roles have not been fully defined.

There are two IL-1 receptors. Upon binding IL-1α or IL-1β, the type I receptor (IL-1RI) binds to the IL-1R accessory protein (IRAP) and transduces a signal. IL-1RII, the type II receptor, is a decoy receptor and competitive inhibitor; both the cell bound and secreted forms of IL-1RII bind with high affinity and avidity to IL-1β but transduce no signal. Of note, IL-1RII binds 50-fold less well to the inhibitory IL-1Ra.

In addition, it has been shown that approximately 20% of the general population have naturally occurring antibodies to IL-1α. It can be hypothesized that the outcome of reactions involving IL-1 depends on the balance of pro-inflammatory (IL-1α, IL-1β) and anti-inflammatory factors (secreted and intracellular IL-1Ra, cell bound and secreted IL-1RII, anti-IL-1 antibodies). That such balance can be of relevance has been demonstrated in inflammatory arthritis [13]. Of note, only

5% of cell surface IL-1RI receptors need to be bound by IL-1 to induce cell activation. Because IL-1Ra is a competitive inhibitor, it must be present in substantial excess to be effective; for example, 10- to 100-fold excess IL-1Ra relative to IL-1β is required to inhibit 50% of IL-1 responses [11,12].

Activities of TNF and IL-1

TNF and IL-1 mediate a myriad of inflammatory and immunoregulatory activities (see Table 1). Not only is there substantial overlap in the activities of these cytokines, but data from *in vitro* studies suggest that TNF and IL-1 may be synergistic in effecting certain functions. The diverse actions mediated by IL-1 and TNF provide the basis for their important role in the pathogenesis of RA (see Table 1).

Although the induction of inflammation mediated by TNF and IL-1 is important to the signs and symptoms of RA, it may also contribute to the immunologic process that drives this chronic disease. It has been suggested that productive immune responses are facilitated by cognate immune interactions that take place in the setting of an active inflammatory milieu [16]. Thus, if sufficient quantities of pro-inflammatory cytokines are released in the course of tissue injury or in response to various stimuli, this may activate antigen presenting cells such as dendritic cells and thereby potentiate autoimmune reactivity. A correlate of this hypothesis would be that inhibition of these cytokines could be immunomodulatory in addition to being anti-inflammatory.

Evidence for a role of TNF and IL-1 in rheumatoid arthritis

While consideration of their pro-inflammatory activities strongly suggests a potential role for TNF and IL-1 in RA, more direct evidence comes from analysis of samples from RA patients and animal models of arthritis.

Table 1. Activities and effects of TNF and IL-1.

Effects on the vasculature

- Up-regulate the expression of endothelial adhesion receptors (ICAM-1, VCAM-1 and E-selectin [CD62E]) via activation of gene transcription factor NF-κB, thus facilitating the recruitment of circulating leukocytes into the inflamed synovium and their activation [14]
- Stimulate angiogenesis, which is critical to the growth and propagation of the rheumatoid synovium
- Alter the normal anti-coagulant function of the endothelium towards pro-coagulant activities (e.g. stimulate tissue factor production, down-modulate thrombomodulin)

Effects on cells

- Activate lymphocytes; increase cytokine release, increase antibody production [*IL-1*], modify CD44 adhesive interactions [*TNF*]
- Promote maturation of dendritic cells and their migration from non-lymphoid tissue into secondary lymphoid organs [*TNF*]
- Activate neutrophils and platelets
- Induce proliferation of synoviocytes and fibroblasts, which contribute to the formation of invasive pannus tissue

Effects on mediators

- Induce synthesis of pro-inflammatory cytokines (e.g. IL-6, GM-CSF)
- TNF can potently stimulate the production of IL-1 (plays a central role in activating an inflammatory response)
- Induce synthesis of key pro-inflammatory chemokines (RANTES, IL-8, MIP-1α, MCP-1)
- Induce other inflammatory mediators: prostaglandins (e.g. PGE_2, by inducing expression of cyclooxygenase-2), leukotrienes, PAF, nitric oxide (TNF stimulates the inducible form of nitric oxide synthase) and reactive oxygen species—the effects of these mediators not only confer many signs and symptoms of inflammation, but also potentiate an inflammatory response
- Induce synthesis of metalloproteinases (e.g. collagenases, gelatinases, stromolysins) that mediate bone and cartilage damage (IL-1 may be more potent in this regard)

Other effects

- Cause signs and symptoms of inflammation, such as pain, fever and cachexia [*TNF*] (associated with many of the notable effects of TNF and IL-1 in RA) [15]
- Decrease the *de novo* synthesis of matrix constituents and facilitate mobilization of calcium from bone ('osteoclast activating factor' activity)
- Modulate apoptosis [*TNF*]

*activities preferentially affected by one cytokine are indicated by brackets and italics
ICAM-1: intercellular cell adhesion molecule-1; VCAM-1: vascular cell adhesion molecule-1; NF-κB: nuclear factor-kappa B; IL-1,-6,-8: interleukin-1,-6,-8; TNF: tumor necrosis factor; GM-CSF: granulocyte-macrophage colony-stimulating factor; MIP-1α: macrophage inflammatory protein-1 alpha; MCP-1: monocyte chemotactic protein-1; PGE_2: prostaglandin E_2; PAF: platelet activating factor

Numerous studies have consistently shown an abundance of immunoreactive TNF-α and IL-1 in the synovial fluid and synovial tissues of RA patients [3-5]. Indeed, the predominance of macrophage produced cytokines (e.g. TNF-α, IL-1 and IL-6) and the relative paucity of T cell associated cytokines (e.g. IL-2) have not only highlighted the contribution of pro-inflammatory cytokines to rheumatoid inflammation, but have also called into question the role T cells play in RA [3]. Increased levels of anti-inflammatory factors, such as soluble forms of the TNF receptors, IL-1Ra and IL-1RII, are also present in the serum and synovial fluid of patients with RA. However, it is presumed that these increased concentrations are still insufficient to overcome the excess pro-inflammatory activity of TNF and IL-1 in arthritis [13]. Of note, the increased levels of IL-1 in synovial fluid have been shown to correlate with clinical, radiologic and histologic parameters of disease in RA patients.

Additional evidence for a potential role of TNF and IL-1 in arthritis comes from animal models such as those with collagen-induced arthritis, adjuvant arthritis and streptococcal cell wall arthritis, which bear semblance to human RA. TNF and IL-1 inhibiting therapies have proven efficacious in these models, attenuating inflammation and reducing joint destruction [17]. In animal models, it has been shown that IL-1 inhibition may have a greater protective effect on bone destruction than TNF inhibition; this may not be the case with RA in humans.

Studies of TNF and IL-1 targeted therapies in patients with rheumatoid arthritis

Agents

A number of studies have evaluated inhibitors of TNF and IL-1 in RA (see Table 2). Almost all of the studies published to date have utilized one of the following agents:

1. a chimeric monoclonal anti-TNF-α antibody (infliximab, Remicade®; previously designated cA2)
2. a recombinant p75TNF-R(CD120b)-Fc fusion protein (etanercept, Enbrel®)
3. a humanized monoclonal anti-TNF-α antibody (CDP571)
4. a fully human monoclonal anti-TNF-α antibody (D2E7)
5. a recombinant IL-1Ra (anakinra)

A number of additional inhibitors are in development.

Trial designs

There are important similarities in the designs of these trials. All have enrolled patients with an established diagnosis of RA who also had active disease. Activity was defined as having some combination of abnormalities on process measures such as elevated numbers of swollen and tender joints, increased concentrations of acute phase reactants (e.g. erythrocyte sedimentation rate [ESR] and serum C-reactive protein [CRP]), functional disability, increased amounts of pain and prolonged early morning stiffness. In addition, most trials have enrolled groups of RA patients that might be considered somewhat refractory, by virtue of long disease duration and failure of several disease-modifying anti-rheumatic drugs (DMARDs). More recently, studies have begun to be conducted in patients with early RA. During the trials, patients were typically allowed to continue stable doses of NSAIDs and prednisone (usually ≤7.5 or 10 mg/day). In some studies, patients with persistent disease activity while on a DMARD (typically methotrexate [MTX]) remained on stable doses of DMARD during the trial.

Efficacy in the trials was usually assessed utilizing composite criteria, such as the American College of Rheumatology (ACR) criteria [18]. Such criteria, which require improvement in multiple variables, are more stringent than analysis of improvement in one or only selected clinical variables. Trials progressed in phases from small, open trials through to large randomized, double-blind, controlled clinical trials. In Table 2, results from these more rigorous types of trials are presented [19-36].

Clinical efficacy (see Table 2)

There are several noteworthy points from these trials. First, the clinical efficacy of these agents is quite remarkable, particularly given the severity of arthritis of the patients enrolled in the trials. For example, although trials typically required six to nine tender and swollen joints for enrollment, actual disease activity of patients beginning the trials often far exceeded these levels. Although many of the trials have been 6 months in length, several of the trials have been longer, or have had extended open label treatment and follow-up. In addition to being effective, therapy was generally well tolerated. Injectable agents have been associated with some local reactions, while intravenous agents have on occasion been associated with mild infusion reactions; however, therapy rarely needed to be interrupted. Some of these studies were published several years ago; therefore, this review will focus on the most relevant recent information for each of these agents.

Infliximab

The first studies testing TNF inhibition in RA were conducted with infliximab. Significant results from early open trials paved the way for a series of larger, double-blind, placebo-controlled trials [19-21]. In the early controlled trials, the efficacy of infliximab was convincingly demonstrated; however, disease activity recurred upon discontinuation of therapy. This, along with the growing safety experience gained with therapy, provided the rationale for studies with longer duration of treatment. In one study, concurrent therapy with methotrexate at a dose of 7.5 mg/week seemed to enhance the clinical response to infliximab and also perhaps to decrease its immunogenicity (as assessed by levels of human anti-chimeric antibodies [HACA]) [21].

Table 2. Published randomized controlled clinical trials of TNF and IL-1 inhibitors in RA.

Agent	Dosage	Concurrent DMARD	Patients	Results/Comments
Infliximab [19]	Single dose of 0, 1 or 10 mg/kg	None	n=73 81% RF+ Mean disease duration: 8 years Mean DMARDs failed: 3.2	Achievement at week 4 of a Paulus 20% response: 10 mg –79%,1 mg–44%, placebo–8% Significant improvement in the anti-TNF groups; extent and duration of response increased with higher dose
Infliximab [20]	Single dose of 0, 5, 10 or 20 mg/kg	MTX 10 mg/week	n=28 82% RF+ Mean disease duration: 6.2 years Mean DMARDs failed: 2.8	Achievement of an ACR 20% response: 14% placebo, 81% infliximab Extent and duration of response dose dependent
Infliximab [21]	0, 1, 3 or 10 mg/kg at weeks 0, 2, 6, 10 and 14	MTX 7.5 mg/week or placebo	n=101 Mean disease duration: 10 years Mean DMARDs failed: 2.4	Concurrent MTX enhanced and prolonged clinical response to infliximab 80% of patients receiving MTX +3 or 10 mg/kg infliximab sustained response through the 26 weeks of the trial
Infliximab [22]	0, 3 or 10 mg/kg every 4 or 8 weeks (initial evaluation 6 months; study continued to 2 years)	MTX ≥12.5 mg/week	n=428 81% RF+ Mean disease duration: 8.4 years 37% had prior joint surgery Mean DMARDs failed (excluding MTX): 2.6	3 and 10 mg/kg given every 4 or 8 weeks had comparable efficacy ACR 20% response 6 months: 20%–placebo, 52%–infliximab ACR 50% response 6 months: 5%–placebo, 28%–infliximab ACR 70% response 6 months: 0%–placebo, 12%–infliximab Efficacy persisted through 54 weeks Treatment improved QOL Treatment arrested progression of structural damage on X-ray (median change Sharp score 0.0 infliximab, +4.0 MTX alone)

Agent	Dosage	Concurrent DMARD	Patients	Results/Comments
CDP571 [23]	Single dose of 0, 0.1, 1 or 10 mg/kg	None	n=36 Mean disease duration: 6 years Mean DMARDs failed: 3.5	Dose dependent improvement in several clinical parameters
Etanercept [24]	0, 2, 4, 8 or 16 mg/m^2 twice weekly x 4 weeks (after loading dose)	None	n=22 (6 assessed for safety only, 16 for safety and efficacy)	Joint and pain scores decreased in 45% of treated patients compared with 22% of placebo
Etanercept [25]	0, 0.25, 2 or 16 mg/m^2 twice weekly x 12 weeks	None	n=180 78% had RA >5 years	ACR 20%: placebo–14%, 0.25 mg/m^2–33%, 2 mg/m^2–46%, 16 mg/m^2–75% ACR 50%: placebo–7%, 0.25 mg/m^2–9%, 2 mg/m^2–22%, 16 mg/m^2–57% Treatment improved QOL
Etanercept [26]	0, 10 or 25 mg twice weekly x 6 months	None	n=234 80% RF+ Mean disease duration: 12 years 90% had failed MTX	ACR 20%: placebo–11%, 10 mg–51%, 25 mg–59% ACR 50%: placebo–5%, 10 mg–24%, 25 mg–40%
Etanercept [27]	0 or 25 mg twice weekly x 6 months	MTX 15–25 mg/week	n=89 86% RF+ Mean disease duration: 13 years Mean DMARDs failed: 2.7	ACR 20%: placebo–27%, etanercept–71% ACR 50%: placebo–3%, etanercept–39% ACR 70%: placebo–0%, etanercept–15%
Etanercept [30]	0.4 mg/kg twice weekly (max dose 25 mg); 3 month open therapy with etanercept followed by 4 month placebo-controlled study	None	n=69 (patients with juvenile chronic arthritis) Mean age 10.5 years Mean disease duration: 6 years 72% on MTX at screening	JRA core set criteria used, flare of disease was primary outcome; in blinded, controlled part of study, 28% of etanercept patients flared, compared to 81% of placebo controls

Agent	Dosage	Concurrent DMARD	Patients	Results/Comments
Etanercept [31]	10 or 25 mg twice weekly x 12 months versus escalating dose of MTX (mean 18.3 mg/week)	None	n=632 87% RF+ (patients required to be RF+ or have X-ray erosion) Early RA (required <3 years, mean 11.5 months) MTX naïve, 42% previously used other DMARD	At 6 months: ACR-N: 25 mg etanercept–38%, MTX–33% Decreased progression in Sharp score: 25 mg etanercept group +0.8, compared to MTX +1.3 or 10 mg etanercept +1.4 Percentage of patients with no new erosions: MTX–57%, 25 mg etanercept–75% At 12 months: ACR-N: 25 mg group–45%, MTX–39%
D2E7 [32]	0, 20, 40 or 80 mg SQ weekly x 6 months (placebo patients change to 40 mg at 3 months)	None	n=283	At 3 months ACR 20% placebo response: 10% and increased to 50% after change to active treatment At 6 months ACR 20% for active groups: 20 mg–56%, 40 mg–64%, 80 mg–63% Treatment may arrest progression in X-ray damage [33]
IL-1Ra [35]	0, 30, 75 or 150 mg/day SQ x 6 months	None	n=472 69% RF+ 75% previously used DMARDs Mean disease duration: 4 years	ACR 20: placebo–27%, 30 mg–39%, 75 mg–34%, 150 mg–43% Change in Larsen (X-ray) score: placebo +6.3, 30 mg +3.5, 75 mg +3.6, 150 mg +3.7
IL-1Ra [36]	0, 0.04, 0.1, 0.4, 1 or 2 mg/kg/day SQ x 6 months	MTX 12.5–25 mg/week	n=419	ACR 20: placebo–23%, 1 mg/kg–42%, 2 mg/kg–35%

ACR: American College of Rheumatology criteria; ACR-N: ACR numeric; ACR 20(%): American College of Rheumatology response criteria representing a 20% improvement from the baseline; DMARDs: disease-modifying anti-rheumatic drugs; RF+: rheumatoid factor positive; JRA: juvenile rheumatoid arthritis; MTX: methotrexate; QOL: quality of life; SQ: subcutaneous; TNF: tumor necrosis factor

Further studies conducted on patients with refractory disease (persistent active RA despite the use of higher doses of methotrexate) supported the impressive efficacy of infliximab [20].

These early studies culminated in the large ATTRACT study [22]. This study proved that addition of infliximab to patients with active disease despite concurrent methotrexate was significantly superior to treatment with methotrexate alone. The initial promising results, from an analysis of responses at 6 months of treatment, have been shown to be sustained through 54 weeks of follow-up [28]. In addition to achieving substantial efficacy as measured by all the usual clinical parameters, the use of infliximab was associated with significant improvement in functional status and quality of life [28]. Perhaps most remarkably, patients receiving infliximab had an arrest of the progression of joint damage as assessed by X-ray change scores. Thus, median change of the Sharp score at 1 year for infliximab treated patients was 0.0 units (mean change +0.55; baseline score 50.5), indicating essentially no overall progression. The median change in score for patients on methotrexate alone was +4.0 units (mean change +7.0; baseline score 55.5); this amount of progression is roughly what would have been predicted given the severity of patients' disease [28,29]. These results are exceptional; while previously RA patients responding clinically to therapy with various DMARDs have had a slowing rate of change on X-ray, no therapy heretofore available has been shown to prevent progression of structural damage to this extent.

Etanercept

Etanercept was the first TNF inhibitor to receive USA Food and Drug Administration (FDA) approval for clinical use in RA. Approval was based on the results of a number of studies showing the efficacy of etanercept either alone or in conjunction with methotrexate in over 500 patients with RA (see Table 2) [24–27]. Initial studies established the efficacy of etanercept and also the optimal dose of 25 mg twice weekly (corresponding to the 16 mg/m^2 used in some studies) [24,25]. Although efficacy was impressive, disease activity recurred upon discontinuation of treatment, prompting longer term treatment paradigms. Many patients from these early trials have continued in long-term open label follow-up. In addition to improving clinical parameters of disease, etanercept was also shown to improve quality of life measures [26]. A trial of etanercept in patients with active RA despite concurrent methotrexate has also been performed; the efficacy of etanercept in such patients was again impressive [27].

Since approval, etanercept has been widely used in clinical practice and its effectiveness in these situations is similar to the substantial efficacy demonstrated in clinical trials. Based on the promising results of a clinical trial of 69 patients, etanercept has been approved for the therapy of juvenile chronic arthritis (previously known as juvenile rheumatoid arthritis, or JRA) [30].

In addition, a large trial of etanercept in patients with early RA was recently completed. In that trial, the efficacy of two doses of etanercept (10 or 25 mg twice weekly) was compared with an accelerated dosing of methotrexate (mean dose MTX 18.3 mg/week within 8 weeks) in MTX naïve RA patients with less than 3 years of disease [31]. The higher dose of etanercept had a more rapid onset of action, yielding a significant difference versus methotrexate by area-under-the-curve analysis. Moreover, although the rate of X-ray progression appeared to be slowed by both agents, the effect of 25 mg etanercept was greater than that of methotrexate (mean change in Sharp scores: MTX +1.3 units, 10 mg etanercept +1.4 units, 25 mg etanercept +0.8 units). The number of patients developing new erosions was also fewer among patients in the 25 mg etanercept group.

CDP571

Results from a controlled study of the humanized anti-TNF-α antibody CDP571 are shown in Table 2. Although efficacy was seen with this agent, the extent of response may have been somewhat less than that achieved with other anti-TNF-α antibodies (e.g. infliximab). No further studies of this agent have been conducted recently.

D2E7

D2E7 is a fully human monoclonal antibody to TNF-α. Even though human protein can elicit an immune response, a fully human agent could offer advantages over agents with foreign (e.g. murine) components as regards immunogenicity, and hence tolerability and long-term efficacy. D2E7 is undergoing assessment in a number of trials. Preliminary results from several studies are available. In a double-blind, placebo-controlled, randomized Phase II trial, 283 patients were treated with placebo or one of three doses of D2E7 (20, 40 or 80 mg) by weekly subcutaneous injection for 6 months (placebo patients switched to active treatment at 3 months) [32]. Clinical results were impressive, with an ACR 20 response of 10% for placebo patients compared to approximately 60% for D2E7 treated patients. Efficacy was comparable among the doses. At present, several doses and dosing regimens are under investigation. Interestingly, analysis of X-rays for a subset of patients receiving D2E7 suggests that this therapy may be able to arrest progression of structural damage, as evidenced by complete inhibition of X-ray score changes [33]. If these results are borne out, it would offer additional support to the results noted with infliximab.

IL-1Ra

Recombinant human IL-1Ra has been utilized in several RA trials. In an early controlled (but not placebo-controlled) trial, three different doses (20, 70 or 200 mg) and three dose schedules (one, three or seven times weekly) of IL-1Ra followed by weekly maintenance dosing were assessed [34]. Without a placebo or other comparison group it is hard to assess efficacy, but daily administration (as opposed to less frequent) and higher doses of IL-1Ra seemed more effective. A placebo-controlled trial of daily dosing with 0, 30, 75 or 150 mg IL-1Ra has been reported [35]. Clinical responses were dose-dependent, with the greatest response in the highest dose group. A slowing of X-ray damage was noted with IL-1Ra compared to placebo and it was comparable among the three active treatment groups. Another placebo-controlled trial has assessed the effect of daily doses (0, 0.04, 0.1, 0.4, 1.0 or 2.0 mg/kg/day) of IL-1Ra in RA patients with active disease despite concurrent MTX [36]. In this study, dose-dependent clinical efficacy was again demonstrated, with optimal efficacy at the 1 mg/kg/day dose.

Adverse effects

Perhaps the most important adverse effects that might potentially be observed with inhibitors of the key pro-inflammatory cytokines TNF and IL-1 are risk of infection and malignancy. In addition, there may be less serious untoward reactions to these inhibitors that may relate to the particular agent utilized (e.g. infusion or local reactions). With TNF inhibitors, development of intermittent positive test for autoantibodies (e.g. anti-DNA), which do not appear to be associated with the development of clinical disease, appears to be a predictable (i.e. approximately 10% of treated patients) but not particularly serious phenomenon.

Infection

TNF and IL-1 mediate a myriad of activities relevant to normal inflammation and immunity (see Table 1) as they serve a central role in host defense. Therefore, increased susceptibility to infections is a potential concern when utilizing these inhibitors. Complicating the analysis of any treatment-related increased risk of infection is the heightened predilection RA patients have for infections, irrespective of treatment [37]. Of note, the subset of RA patients with the greatest susceptibility to infection (i.e. those with severe, active disease) have also been the type of patient most commonly enrolled in trials of these agents. In RA trials, a number of infections have occurred among patients receiving TNF and IL-1 inhibitors. However, these infections seemed to respond to appropriate antimicrobial therapy and most did not become serious (i.e. require hospitalization or intravenous therapies). In post-marketing surveillance of approximately 25,000 RA patients treated with etanercept after it had been approved for use in the USA, 30 serious infections including six septic deaths were reported. Although this raised concern, the frequency of these outcomes was well within the range that could be expected given the patient population and their severity of disease. Nevertheless, when using TNF and IL-1 inhibitors, holding treatment should be a consideration when there is potential for serious infection.

Malignancy

Immunosurveillance is also critical to the host defense against malignancy. Therefore, there is a theoretical risk of increasing the risk of malignancy with immunomodulatory therapies such as TNF and IL-1 inhibitors. As is the case for infections, patients with RA also appear to have an increased susceptibility to certain malignancies, particularly lymphoproliferative cancers [37–39]. This risk must be kept in mind when evaluating results and implying causality in therapeutic trials. In trials of the various TNF inhibitors in RA patients, several cases of hematologic and other malignancies have been reported. At present, it does not appear that the number of cancers observed significantly exceeds the rate that would be expected in this population.

Encouraging data regarding the risks for development of serious infections, malignancies and other severe outcomes have come from longer term observation of patients treated in clinical trials of infliximab and etanercept [40,41]. Although vigilance in the treatment of individual patients is indicated, and longer term observational studies would provide critical information, at present it does not appear that these agents induce substantial clinically relevant immunosuppression or an increase in susceptibility to serious infections or malignancy.

Antigenicity

Considerations of antigenicity are germane to any biologic therapy. Development of antibodies to a therapeutic agent could diminish its serum half-life, decrease efficacy and cause adverse reactions. Various factors affect the immunogenicity of foreign antigens, including the degree of antigenic variation or 'foreignness'; dose (both high and low doses of an antigen are capable of inducing tolerance); route of administration (cutaneous administration is more likely to induce antibody responses than intravenous or oral administration); frequency of treatment (continuous therapy is less immunogenic then intermittent therapy); and immunomodulatory effects of the agent itself or of concurrent treatment (immunosuppressive agents can decrease immunogenicity). The extent of reactivity to TNF and IL-1 inhibitors and the clinical implications of this reactivity will be an important area of research as these agents gain wider clinical use.

Potential differences between TNF inhibitors

As noted, several different TNF inhibitors have been studied in RA patients. Definitive comparison of these agents can only come from head-to-head comparison studies; such studies are unlikely in the near future. However, clinical efficacy achieved with the various agents appears to be comparable. Nevertheless, there are potentially important differences among the agents, for example:

1. the anti-TNF-α monoclonal antibodies are specific for TNF-α; soluble TNF receptor constructs bind both TNF-α and LT-α

2. all agents bind TNF with high affinity, whereas monoclonal antibodies may have a higher avidity

Whether any of these differences is associated with differential efficacy or toxicity, remains to be demonstrated. Importantly, a number of TNF inhibitors under development have distinct pharmacodynamic and pharmacokinetic characteristics compared to the agents already considered; how this may affect their efficacy and safety remains to be determined.

Future directions

Given the extraordinary efficacy and clinical effectiveness that have been demonstrated with inhibitors of TNF and IL-1, there are a number of exciting avenues for future development of these agents. Three of the most eagerly awaited developments include:

1. optimizing the use of currently available inhibitors

2. the introduction of novel agents

3. the potential for combination therapy

Optimizing the use of currently available inhibitors

There are several avenues that could facilitate optimal utilization of TNF and IL-1 inhibitors in RA. Perhaps the most immediately relevant area of research would be the delineation of those subsets of patients for whom these therapies are most effective and safest. In animal studies, it has been shown that TNF and IL-1 inhibitors may be more or less effective at different stages of arthritis [17]. In RA, it has also been suggested that patients may be heterogeneous in their clinical presentations as well as their response to certain therapeutics. Almost all earlier studies of these inhibitors have been in patients with refractory established RA; whether the responses in patients with earlier disease or other subsets of patients will be distinct is under investigation.

Although TNF inhibitors have been effective for the majority of treated patients, only a subset of patients achieve remission or near remission; moreover, a minority of patients have minimal if any response. The ability prospectively to identify subsets of RA patients who could be expected to have exceptional efficacy yet minimal toxicity would be a tremendous breakthrough. To date, simple clinical characteristics (e.g. age, sex, rheumatoid factor [RF] status, disease activity at initiation, etc.) do not seem to allow identification of subsequent responses.

Given the observation that there can be heterogeneity of cytokine expression in synovial biopsy specimens, some measure of local cytokine activity may provide clinically relevant information. Perhaps most intriguingly, allelic polymorphisms in genes encoding TNF, IL-1 and other cytokines have been noted. Preliminary results suggest that such genetic variation may be relevant to disease outcome in RA [42]; this may provide critical insights into optimal therapeutic strategies.

Other methods of inhibiting TNF and IL-1

Besides the therapies described above, additional inhibitors of TNF (e.g. a soluble p55 TNF receptor) and IL-1 (soluble form of the IL-1RI) are being assessed in early clinical trials. These approaches have in common the involvement of macromolecules. While they are specific and effective, inherent limitations of macromolecules include their large size (which can enhance immunogenicity and affect pharmacodynamics) and high cost (they are complicated biologic agents which require exacting production standards). It should be noted parenthetically that, although the costs of these agents are substantial, determination of their potential cost-efficacy must take into account the extent of clinical response associated with therapy, as well as their effects on quality of life and long-term damage [43]. There are potential solutions for some of these concerns with macromolecules; for example, generating agents in transgenic plants or animals, or synthesizing constructs with targeted delivery systems.

A tremendous effort has already been undertaken to develop novel small molecule inhibitors of TNF and IL-1 that could be as effective yet cheaper than current agents and perhaps even orally available. Some examples of potential agents include inhibitors of TACE and ICE (which cleave these cytokines from the cell surface), inhibitors of phosphodiesterase IV (which regulates TNF-α production), inhibitors of NF-κB, peptidomimetic inhibitors of cytokine-receptor interaction and gene transfer to over-express TNF and IL-1 receptors [44-46]. These are areas of intense investigation and development.

Combination therapy with cytokine inhibitors

There are a number of potential advantages of combination therapy in RA (see Table 3). Additive efficacy would be an increase in the extent of response or number of responders compared to single agent therapy. Synergistic efficacy implies that the extent of response is more than the additive effects of both agents when used as monotherapy. This might be achieved by a combination of agents with similar mechanisms, or by agents with distinct targets and actions (see Table 4). If enhanced efficacy were achieved, the doses of agents required to be used might be lessened, which could

---

Table 3. Potential benefits of combination therapy in RA.

- Additive efficacy
- Synergistic efficacy
- Reduced toxicity
- Greater immunomodulation

Table 4. Possible combinations of biologic/cytokine targeted therapies.

Anti-inflammatory + anti-inflammatory

- TNF inhibitor + IL-1 inhibitor
- TNF or IL-1 inhibitor + IL-10
- TNF or IL-1 inhibitor + chemokine inhibitor

Anti-inflammatory + immunomodulator

- TNF or IL-1 inhibitor + IL-2 inhibitor
- TNF or IL-1 inhibitor + IL-12 or IL-18 inhibitor, or IL-4
- TNF or IL-1 inhibitor + non-depleting anti-CD4 antibody
- TNF or IL-1 inhibitor + angiogenesis inhibitor

---

then reduce the risk of adverse effects. For example, a combination of doses of agents that were each suboptimal when given alone might be safer yet more effective when used together. In addition, by targeting distinct components of the immune response, combinations of agents might achieve greater immunomodulation. A potential benefit of this could be decreased immunogenicity of biologic agents.

To date, TNF inhibitors have been used primarily in combination with methotrexate. The efficacy and tolerability of these agents with other DMARDs (e.g. leflunomide, cyclosporine, sulfasalazine) need to be assessed in RA. Perhaps more intriguing would be the combination of cytokine inhibitors, or the combination of cytokine inhibitors and other biologic agents (see Table 4). Using such combinations, there have been striking results in animal models, with synergistic efficacy in reducing inflammation and even complete inhibition of bone destruction [47–49]. Similar approaches may be expected to be assessed in RA patients in the near future.

Conclusions

Treatment of RA patients with TNF and IL-1 inhibitors has proven to be extremely effective. Rigorous studies and increasing clinical experience have proven the utility and acceptability of these agents. Larger, long-term studies will help further define their effectiveness and safety. Additional studies have begun to define the optimal treatment paradigms for the use of TNF and IL-1 inhibitors, including combination therapy. This should afford tangible and substantial clinical benefit to some of the patients suffering from this aggressive disease. Further developments in this area can be expected to allow the clinician to refine and optimize therapy with these agents.

References

1. Sewell KL, Trentham DE. Pathogenesis of rheumatoid arthritis. Lancet 1993;341:283–6.
2. Kavanaugh A, Lipsky P. Rheumatoid arthritis. In: Rich R (Ed). Clinical Immunology; Principles and Practice. New York: Mosby, 1996. 1093–116.
3. Firestein GS, Zvaifler NJ. How important are T cells in chronic rheumatoid synovitis? Arthritis Rheum 1990;33:768–73.
4. Koch AE, Kunkel SL, Strieter RM. Cytokines in rheumatoid arthritis. J Investig Med 1995;43:28–38.
5. Feldmann M, Brennan FM, Maini RN. Role of cytokines in rheumatoid arthritis. Annu Rev Immunol 1996;14:397–440.
6. Firestein G, Zvaifler N. Anticytokine therapy in rheumatoid arthritis. N Engl J Med 1997;337:195–7.
7. Arend WP, Dayer JM. Inhibition of the production and effects of interleukin-1 and tumor necrosis factor alpha in rheumatoid arthritis. Arthritis Rheum 1995;38:151–60.
8. Bazzoni F, Beutler B. The tumor necrosis factor ligand and receptor families. N Engl J Med 1996;334:1717–25.
9. Sacca R, Cuff C, Lesslauer W et al. Differential activities of secreted lymphotoxin-alpha3 and membrane lymphotoxin-alpha1beta2 in lymphotoxin-induced inflammation: critical role of TNF receptor 1 signaling. J Immunol 1998;160:485–91.
10. Darnay BG, Aggarwal BB. Signal transduction by tumor necrosis factor and tumor necrosis factor related ligands and their receptors. Ann Rheum Dis 1999;58(Suppl. 1):I2–I13.
11. Dinarello CA. Biologic basis for interleukin-1 in disease. Blood 1996;87:2095–147.

12. Rosenwasser LJ. Biologic activities of IL-1 and its role in human disease. J Allergy Clin Immunol 1998;102:344–50.

13. Miller LC, Lynch EA, Isa S et al. Balance of synovial fluid IL-1 beta and IL-1 receptor antagonist and recovery from Lyme arthritis. Lancet 1993;341:146–8.

14. Kavanaugh A. Antiadhesion therapy in rheumatoid arthritis: A review of recent progress. BioDrugs 1997;7:119–33.

15. Dinarello CA, Cannon JG, Wolff SM et al. Tumor necrosis factor (cachetin) is an endogenous pyrogen and induces production of interleukin 1. J Exp Med 1986;163:1433–50.

16. Benoist C, Mathis D. Autoimmunity. The pathogen connection. Nature 1998;394:227–8.

17. Joosten LA, Helsen MM, van de Loo FA et al. Anticytokine treatment of established type II collagen-induced arthritis in DBA/1 mice. A comparative study using anti-TNF-alpha, anti-IL-1 alpha/beta and IL-1Ra. Arthritis Rheum 1996;39:797–809.

18. Felson DT, Anderson JN, Boers M et al. American College of Rheumatology. Preliminary definition of improvement in rheumatoid arthritis. Arthritis Rheum 1995;38:727–35.

19. Elliott MJ, Maini RN, Feldmann M. Randomized double-blind comparison of chimeric monoclonal antibody to tumor necrosis factor alpha (cA2) versus placebo in rheumatoid arthritis. Lancet 1994;344:1105–10.

20. Kavanaugh A, St Clair EW, McCune WJ et al. Chimeric anti-tumor necrosis factor-alpha monoclonal antibody treatment of patients with rheumatoid arthritis receiving methotrexate therapy. J Rheumatol 2000;27:841–50.

21. Maini RN, Breedveld FC, Kalden JR et al. Therapeutic efficacy of multiple intravenous infusions of anti-tumor necrosis factor-alpha monoclonal antibody combined with low-dose weekly methotrexate in rheumatoid arthritis. Arthritis Rheum 1998;41:1552–63.

22. Maini R, St Clair EW, Breedveld F et al. Infliximab (chimeric anti-tumor necrosis factor-alpha monoclonal antibody) versus placebo in rheumatoid arthritis patients receiving concomitant methotrexate: a randomised phase III trial. Lancet 1999;354:1932–9.

23. Rankin ECC, Choy EHS, Kassimos D et al. The therapeutic effects of an engineered human anti-tumor necrosis factor antibody (CDP571) in rheumatoid arthritis. Br J Rheumatol 1995;34:334–42.

24. Moreland LW, Margolies G, Heck LW et al. Recombinant soluble tumor necrosis factor receptor (p80) fusion protein: toxicity and dose finding trial in refractory rheumatoid arthritis. J Rheumatol 1996;23:1849–55.

25. Moreland LW, Baumgartner SW, Schiff MH et al. Treatment of rheumatoid arthritis with a recombinant human tumor necrosis factor receptor (p75)-Fc fusion protein. N Engl J Med 1997;337:141–7.

26. Moreland LW, Schiff MH, Baumgartner SW et al. Etanercept therapy in rheumatoid arthritis. A randomized controlled trial. Ann Intern Med 1999;130:478–86.

27. Weinblatt ME, Kremer JM, Bankhurst AD et al. A trial of etanercept, a recombinant tumor necrosis factor receptor:Fc fusion protein, in patients with rheumatoid arthritis receiving methotrexate. N Engl J Med 1999;340:253–9.

28. Emery P, Maini R, Lipsky PE et al. Infliximab plus methotrexate prevents structural damage, reduces signs and symptoms and improves disability in patients with active early rheumatoid arthritis. Ann Rheum Dis 2000;59 (Suppl. I):48.

29. van der Heijde, Emery P, Lipsky PE et al. Consistent improvement in radiographic joint damage in patients with active rheumatoid arthritis treated with infliximab along with methotrexate. Ann Rheum Dis 2000;59(Suppl. I):161.

30. Lovell D, Giannini E, Whitmore J et al. Safety and efficacy of tumor necrosis factor receptor p75 Fc fusion protein (TNFR:Fc; Enbrel) in polyarticular course juvenile rheumatoid arthritis. Arthritis Rheum 1998;41(Suppl. I):S130.

31. Martin R, Ruderman E, Fleischmann R et al. A phase III trial of etanercept vs methotrexate (MTX) in early rheumatoid arthritis (Enbrel ERA trial). Ann Rheum Dis 2000;59 (Suppl. I):47.

32. van de Putte LBA, Rau R, Breedveld FC et al. Six month efficacy of the fully human anti-TNF antibody D2E7 in rheumatoid arthritis. Ann Rheum Dis 2000;59 (Suppl. I):48.

33. Rau R, Herborn G, Sander O et al. Long-term treatment with the fully human anti-TNF antibody D2E7 in rheumatoid arthritis – effects on radiographic disease progression and pro-MMPs. Ann Rheum Dis 2000;59 (Suppl. I):48.

34. Campion GV, Lebsack ME, Lookbaugh J et al. Dose-range and dose-frequency study of recombinant human interleukin-1 receptor antagonist in patients with rheumatoid arthritis. The IL-Ra Study Group. Arthritis Rheum 1996;39:1092–101.

35. Bresnihan B, Alvaro-Gracia JM, Cobby M et al. Treatment of rheumatoid arthritis with recombinant human interleukin-1 receptor antagonist. Arthritis Rheum 1998;41:2196–204.

36. Cohen S, Hurd EE, Cush JJ et al. Treatment of interleukin-1 receptor antagonist in combination with methotrexate in rheumatoid arthritis patients. Ann Rheum Dis 2000;59 (Suppl. I):150.

37. Wolfe F, Mitchell DM, Sibley JT et al. The mortality of rheumatoid arthritis. Arthritis Rheum 1994;37:481–94.

38. Cibere J, Sibley J, Haga M. Rheumatoid arthritis and the risk of malignancy. Arthritis Rheum 1997;40:1580–6.

39. Gridley G, McLaughlin JK, Ekbom A et al. Incidence of cancer among patients with rheumatoid arthritis. J Natl Cancer Inst 1993;85:307–11.

40. Kavanaugh A, Schaible T, DeWoody K et al. Long-term follow-up of patients treated with infliximab (anti-TNF-alpha monoclonal antibody) in clinical trials. Arthritis Rheum 1999;42(Suppl.):S401.

41. Moreland LW, Cohen SB, Baumgartner S et al. Long-term use of etanercept in patients with DMARD refractory rheumatoid arthritis. Arthritis Rheum 1999;42(Suppl.):S401.

42. Mattey DL, Hassell AB, Dawes PT et al. Interaction between tumor necrosis factor microsatellite polymorphisms and the HLA-DRB1 shared epitope in rheumatoid arthritis: influence on disease outcome. Arthritis Rheum 1999;42:2698–704.

43. Kavanaugh A, Heudebert G, Cush J et al. Cost evaluation of novel therapeutics in rheumatoid arthritis (CENTRA): a decision analysis model. Semin Arthritis Rheum 1996;25:297–307.

44. Black RA, Rauch CT, Kozlosky CJ et al. A metalloproteinase disintegrin that releases tumor necrosis factor-α from cells. Nature 1997;385:729–33.

45. Le CH, Nicolson AG, Morales et al. Suppression of collagen-induced arthritis through adenovirus-mediated transfer of a modified tumor necrosis factor alpha receptor gene. Arthritis Rheum 1997;40:1662–9.

46. Takasaki W, Kajino Y, Kajino K et al. Structure-based design and characterization of exocyclic peptidomimetics that inhibit TNFα binding to its receptor. Nat Biotechnol 1997;15:1266–70.

47. Bendele AM, Chilpala ES, Scherrer J et al. Combination benefit to treatment with the cytokine inhibitors interleukin-1 receptor antagonist (IL-1Ra) and soluble tumor necrosis factor type I (sTNF-RI) in animal models of rheumatoid arthritis. Arthritis Rheum (in press).

48. Kim KN, Watanabe S, Ma Y et al. Viral IL-10 and soluble TNF receptor act synergistically to inhibit collagen-induced arthritis following adenovirus-mediated gene transfer. J Immunol 2000;164:1576–81.

49. Marinova-Mutafchieva L, Williams RO, Mauri C et al. A comparative study into the mechanisms of action of anti-tumor necrosis factor α, anti-CD4 and combined anti-tumor necrosis factor α/anti-CD4 treatment in early collagen-induced arthritis. Arthritis Rheum 2000;43:638–44.

6

Emerging therapies for rheumatoid arthritis

Mark C Genovese and William H Robinson

Rheumatoid arthritis (RA) is characterized by chronic inflammatory synovitis, formation of pannus and erosive joint destruction. Although the etiology of the inflammatory response remains elusive, RA is known to be mediated by T cells, B cells and macrophages. It is hypothesized that an autoimmune T cell response induces production of tumor necrosis factor-α (TNF-α) which drives the inflammatory synovitis and erosive joint destruction [1]. However, anti-TNF-α therapy, like other disease-modifying anti-rheumatic drugs (DMARDs), is not curative and synovitis rapidly returns following its discontinuation. There is tremendous clinical need for more fundamental therapeutic approaches.

Promising novel therapeutic approaches for RA are directed at termination of the underlying autoimmune process and blocking mediators of joint destruction (see Figure 1). These include:

1. peptide- and T cell receptor-based strategies for inactivating or eliminating autoreactive T cells
2. cytokine-based strategies for inducing immune-deviation
3. co-stimulatory molecule blockade
4. therapeutic gene delivery (such as IL-1 receptor antagonist cDNA)
5. blockade of mediators of synovitis and joint destruction

Peptide therapies for rheumatoid arthritis

Peptide-based therapies have the potential to tolerize the immune system by eliminating or inactivating autoreactive

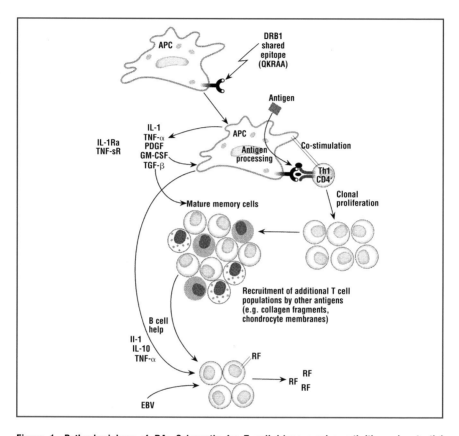

Figure 1. Pathophysiology of RA: Schematic for T cell-driven erosive arthritis and potential therapeutic targets. Antigen is taken up by antigen presenting cells (APCs), proteolytically processed into peptides, and then major histocompatibility complex (MHC):peptide complexes are formed. The MHC:peptide complexes are presented on the surface of the APCs to potentially autoreactive T cells. The DRB1 shared epitope is associated with increased likelihood of developing RA. MHC molecules containing the shared epitope are believed to efficiently bind antigenic self-peptides that activate autoreactive T cells in RA. A co-stimulatory signal is required for T cell activation (see Figure 2). T cell activation results in production of TNF-α by macrophages. TNF-α drives a cascade of inflammatory cytokines, including interleukin-1 (IL-1), IL-6 and granulocyte-macrophage colony-stimulating factor (GM-CSF), that cause inflammatory synovitis and erosive arthritis. Memory T cells are formed and the inflammatory synovitis may be perpetuated by other antigens (e.g. collagen fragments, chondrocyte membranes) and stimuli (e.g. infections and non-specific joint irritation). Potential targets for therapeutic intervention include preventing activation of autoreactive T cells and inhibiting the mediators of the inflammatory synovitis and erosive arthritis. (Schematic reproduced with permission from Harris ED, editor. Rheumatoid Arthritis. Philadelphia: Saunders WB, 1997 [1].)

T cells. However, major histocompatibility complex (MHC):peptide complexes and T cell receptor-peptide vaccines have not shown substantial efficacy, and all other peptide-based therapies are still in preclinical development.

MHC:peptide complexes

Attempts have been made to induce immune tolerance by modulating signals delivered through the T cell receptor (TCR). In RA, the presentation of antigenic self-peptides to autoreactive T cells is presumed to be either an initiating event or a process through which an aberrant immune response is perpetuated.

One therapeutic strategy involves induction of T cell anergy (unresponsiveness) through administration of soluble MHC class II:self-peptide complexes that deliver tolerizing signals to autoreactive T cells. Such MHC:peptide complexes can interact with the TCR in a manner that induces T cell anergy or apoptosis in the absence of co-stimulatory signals, and have demonstrated efficacy in rodent models.

A peptide postulated to be one of the autoantigens involved in the development of RA has been derived from human cartilage glycoprotein 39 (HCgp39). The peptide is under investigation for the treatment of RA as part of a complex containing the MHC molecule HLA-DR4 (B1*0401) [2,3]. This soluble complex (AG4263) was examined in a Phase I study involving patients who had failed at least one DMARD and had active disease despite concomitant use of methotrexate. Patients were randomized to receive one of seven intravenous doses of AG4263 (n=24) or placebo (n=7) over 6 weeks. Preliminary results suggested that out of 157 patients screened, 45 were positive for HLA-DR4 (28.7%) and that 30% of the samples assayed showed T cell reactivity to the peptide derived from HCgp39. The infusions were well tolerated [2]. Sixteen of the 18 patients treated with the highest dosages (60 and 150 µg/kg) achieved a Paulus 20 (20% improvement in at least four out of six core set variables defined by Paulus criteria for severity of RA) compared to four out of seven patients in the placebo cohort [3].

Potential shortcomings of MHC:peptide complexes include the limited prevalence of HCgp39 as a dominant autoantigen in RA, expression of HLA-DR4 by only a fraction of RA patients and unclear efficacy of MHC:peptide therapy in diversified autoimmune responses.

T cell receptor-peptide vaccines

In rodents, collagen-induced arthritis (CIA) is mediated by T cells expressing a limited set of TCR variable (V) gene segments. Injection of peptides derived from the dominant V region(s) triggers an immune response against the pathogenic T cells resulting in elimination of those T cells. A randomized, placebo-controlled, Phase II trial treated 99 RA patients with a T cell receptor-peptide vaccine containing a combination of three peptides derived from Vβ3, Vβ14 and Vβ17 [4]. A trend towards improvement in the groups receiving the T cell receptor-derived peptides was seen.

In a second Phase II study, two different T cell receptor peptide vaccines derived from Vβ3, Vβ14 and Vβ17 were compared in a double-blind randomized placebo-controlled study of 6 months' duration. There was a trend toward improvement in those patients receiving vaccination, particularly those having had the disease for less than 3 years and those on less than 7.5 mg/day of prednisone. In virtually all the treatment groups improvement was seen following three injections, but this had waned by week 20 [5].

Given the heterogeneity of human autoimmune responses in RA, with different patients utilizing different combinations of T cell receptor V gene segments, T cell receptor-peptide-based therapeutics are only likely to possess efficacy for a subset of RA patients. Such constraints, combined with their modest efficacy, diminish enthusiasm for wide-scale use of such a strategy.

Cytokine-based therapeutic strategies

Cytokines play two important roles in the pathophysiology of RA:

1. evidence from animal models suggests that pro-inflammatory cytokines, such as TNF-α, can drive synovitis and erosive joint destruction independent of an ongoing autoimmune response [6]

2. cytokines influence the generation of the specific types of CD4+ helper T cell response, i.e. Th1 versus Th2. Th1 immune responses, characterized by CD4+ T cells that produce interleukin-2 (IL-2), IL-12 and interferon-γ (IFN-γ), are capable of tissue destruction and are associated with autoimmune disease. Th2 CD4+ T cells produce IL-4 and IL-5 which are associated with protection against autoimmunity

There is growing evidence that Th1-like immune responses may, in part, propagate human rheumatoid arthritis. Thus, a proposed treatment strategy is to deviate the autoimmune response towards the non-pathogenic Th2-type response either by blockade of Th1 cytokines or by direct administration of Th2 cytokines.

Inhibition of IL-12

Studies in murine models have demonstrated that the Th1 cytokine IL-12 plays a central role in mediating CIA [7,8]. Use of a combination of anti-IL-12 plus anti-TNF-α antibodies synergistically suppresses and successfully treats CIA following the onset of clinical disease [9].

Increased levels of IL-12 have been detected in the serum and synovial fluid of patients with RA [10]. Also, there is a case report of a RA patient who had a severe exacerbation of disease after receiving recombinant IL-12 as an experimental therapy for cervical cancer [11]. Studies examining mechanisms to interfere with IL-12 are underway in humans.

Inhibition of IFN-γ

IFN-γ, like IL-12, is a Th1 cytokine that drives activation of cytotoxic T cells. In RA patients, increased synovial fluid levels of IFN-γ and synovial T cell production of IFN-γ are observed and probably foster Th1 cell-mediated erosive joint destruction [12]. Phase I clinical trials examining use of an anti-IFN-γ antibody in human RA patients are in progress.

Administration of IFN-β

Recombinant human IFN-β is approved by the USA Food and Drug Administration (FDA) for the treatment of relapsing-remitting multiple sclerosis [13]. Although its mechanism of action is poorly understood, IFN-β is thought to antagonize the effects of IFN-γ and other pro-inflammatory cytokines, and to down-regulate T cell activity. There is optimism that IFN-β might also be an efficacious therapy for human RA.

Eleven patients with active RA were subcutaneously treated with either placebo or IFN-β three times/week for 12 weeks [14]. After 3 months, four patients had achieved an American College of Rheumatology (ACR 20) response (20% improvement in variables defined by the ACR criteria for severity of RA). Based on immunohistologic analysis of synovial biopsies carried out before and after therapy, there was a significant reduction in T cells in addition to a reduction in expression of matrix metalloproteinase-1 (MMP-1), IL-1β, IL-6 and TNF-α.

Phase II clinical trials using IFN-β for the treatment of RA are in progress.

Inhibition of IL-6

IL-6 has been shown to play an important role both in murine models of RA and in human RA. Elevated levels of both IL-6 and soluble IL-6 receptor are observed in the serum and synovial fluid of patients with RA [15-17].

An open-label pilot study was conducted in five patients with RA to examine daily, intravenous administration of a mouse anti-IL-6 antibody for 10 days [18]. A trend towards clinical improvement was observed for several months following treatment and no adverse events were reported.

Anti-IL-6 receptor antibody is also under examination in RA patients and has been associated with a decrease in rheumatoid factor titers and an overall anti-inflammatory effect [19].

Inhibition of T cell activation by co-stimulatory molecule blockade

T cell activation requires two signals (see Figure 2). The first signal is generated by binding of the TCR with an antigenic peptide complexed with MHC molecules on the surface of an antigen-presenting cell (APC). A second signal, also known as the co-stimulatory signal, is required for T cell activation and is mediated by the co-stimulatory molecules CD40L-CD40 and CD28-B7 (including B7-1 and B7-2, also known as CD80 and CD86). The first signal in the absence of the second signal results in T cell anergy or deletion (i.e. immune tolerance). Therefore, therapies that antagonize the second signal, by blocking CD40L-CD40 and/or CD28-B7 signaling, have the potential to induce immune tolerance and thereby turn off autoimmune responses.

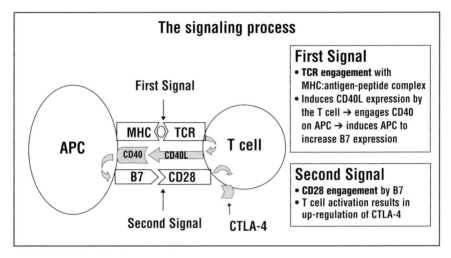

Figure 2. T cell activation requires two signals. The first signal, T cell receptor (TCR) engagement with MHC:antigen-peptide, provides antigen-specificity to the T cell response. The second signal, CD28 engagement by B7 (CD80 and/or CD86), is an essential co-stimulatory signal for T cell activation. The first signal in the absence of the second signal induces T cell tolerance (anergy or deletion). Candidate therapeutic agents including anti-CD40/CD40L, CTLA-4-Ig, and anti-CD80/CD86 all block T cell activation by antagonizing the second signal.

CD40L

Interference with CD40L-CD40 interactions has been shown to reduce the manifestations of autoimmune disease in animal models of systemic lupus erythematosus (SLE), multiple sclerosis, RA and inflammatory bowel disease. Also, treatment with anti-CD40L antibodies at the time of immunization prevents the development of CIA and blocks the development of serum auto-antibodies to collagen, synovial inflammation and joint erosions [20]. Anti-CD40L antibodies may prevent engagement of CD40 on macrophages and synoviocytes, and thereby inhibit their production of pro-inflammatory cytokines, nitric oxide and matrix metalloproteinases. It is thought that activated T cells drive synovial inflammation in RA via CD40L stimulated production of TNF-α.

Anti-CD40L antibody therapy has been utilized in humans for the treatment of other autoimmune diseases including lupus. Two antibody preparations, Biogen-9588 and IDEC-131, have been used in human clinical trials. Biogen-9588 was implicated as a potential cause of thrombo-embolic complications and studies have stopped pending further evaluation. The etiology or pathogenesis of the thrombotic complications is not known.

Different anti-CD40L antibodies may recognize distinct epitopes in the CD40L molecule and both side effects and efficacy may depend on these differences. IDEC-131 has been studied in human Phase I and II clinical trials investigating treatment for SLE. No association with thrombo-embolic complications was reported. It is anticipated that anti-CD40L antibody could be used in the future for the treatment of RA. It has the potential to result in potent anti-inflammatory and disease-modifying effects. However, the long-term safety of this approach is unclear.

CD40

CD40 is expressed on the surface of APCs, including B cells, activated macrophages and synoviocytes. Engagement of CD40 by CD40L leads to a host of downstream changes including T cell co-stimulation, cytotoxic T lymphocyte priming, up-regulation of B cell co-stimulatory molecules (B7-1 and B7-2), promotion of B cell differentiation, germinal center formation, B cell responsiveness to T cell cytokines and immunoglobulin class switching.

In patients with RA, CD40 is expressed on rheumatoid synovial pannus and fibroblasts. It appears that CD40 is involved in chronic activation of RA synovial monocytes. Interference with ligation of the CD40 receptor after administration of anti-CD40 antibodies can inhibit secretion of TNF-α from RA synovial monocytes [21]. Blockade of the

CD40L-CD40 interaction results in deletion of rheumatoid factor-producing B cells.

Clinical trials using anti-CD40 antibodies are underway in humans. It is hoped that CD40-CD40L blockade will lead to the induction of immune tolerance and cause a significant reduction in autoimmune and inflammatory disease, although the safety and efficacy of this approach remain to be established.

B7

B7-1 and B7-2 (CD80 and CD86 are collectively referred to as B7) represent inducible co-stimulatory molecules expressed on the surface of APCs. They bind CD28, found on the surface of T cells. As mentioned previously, engagement of B7 with CD28 (second signal), in conjunction with simultaneous signaling through the TCR (first signal), results in T cell activation (see Figure 2). B7 plays a critical role in the induction of autoimmune arthritis in rodents and represents an important therapeutic target for human RA.

In humans, B7-CD28-mediated cellular interactions between the synovium and infiltrating T cells are associated with the development of synovial inflammation [22]. Both B7-1 and B7-2 are expressed within rheumatoid synovium. However, B7-2 is present in much higher levels than B7-1 [23-25]. This suggests that B7-2 may be the preferred target, although inhibition of both molecules has been necessary for treatment efficacy in animal models of RA [26]. Clinical trials have been designed to utilize anti-B7-1 and anti-B7-2 antibodies both individually and collectively for the treatment of RA in humans.

Cytotoxic T lymphocyte-associated antigen (CTLA-4)

CTLA-4 is a regulatory molecule expressed on the surface of helper T cells following activation. Expression of CTLA-4 blocks excitatory co-stimulatory signals by binding B7 and preventing its binding to CD28, and delivers inhibitory signals to T cells [27]. It is thought that expression of CTLA-4 acts to attenuate T cell responses following activation, so that overactive T cell responses do not develop. Thus, CTLA-4 serves as an inhibitory regulatory checkpoint during T cell activation.

A fusion protein, CTLA-4-Ig, has been designed to block co-stimulation. The protein consists of the extracellular portion of CTLA-4 joined to the Fc portion of IgG. In rat models, CTLA-4-Ig prevents induction of CIA and also reduces the severity of established disease [26,28]. In a small Phase I study in humans with psoriasis, CTLA-4-Ig led to a 50% clinical improvement in disease activity [29]. A Phase II study has been completed in humans examining the safety and efficacy of CTLA-4-Ig in the treatment of RA and results are expected soon.

Gene therapy

Although still in its infancy, gene therapy is a promising treatment strategy for RA that offers the potential to deliver therapeutic proteins to selected anatomic sites. In the first human clinical trial of gene therapy for arthritis, synovial fibroblasts were stably transduced with a retrovirus expressing IL-1 receptor antagonist cDNA [30,31]. Transduced or control autologous fibroblasts were transferred into metacarpal phalangeal joints (MCP) of nine postmenopausal women in a double-blind dose escalation fashion. One week after gene transfer, the MCP joints were surgically removed. All joints receiving the transgene showed evidence of gene expression, and curiously a number of adjacent joints receiving control cells also showed evidence of gene expression. No adverse events were reported with follow-up extending beyond 3 years in several patients. However, the detection of transgene expression in control joints highlights a lack of understanding regarding migration of cells and viruses, and represents just one of the many potential impediments to implementation of such therapy in the clinic [30-32]. Furthermore, given the recent human deaths associated with adenovirus-based gene therapies [33], careful evaluation of potential therapeutics is essential.

Therapeutic modulation of mediators of inflammatory arthritis

p38 inhibition

Another of the promising pathways being explored for possible therapeutic intervention in RA is that of the stress-activated protein kinases (SAPKs) and mitogen-activated protein kinases (MAPKs). Inflammatory stimuli trigger a cascade beginning with cell membrane receptors that activate kinases leading to increased expression of cytokines and growth factors that produce further inflammation and immune activation [34]. p38 is one such protein kinase. Activation of p38 inducibly up-regulates TNF-α, IL-1, IL-6, IL-8, nitric oxide production and cyclooxygenase-2 expression. Inhibition of p38 down-regulates these pro-inflammatory products, but may not result in immune suppression because only inducible, and not constitutive, production is affected. The p38 MAPK inhibitors have demonstrated efficacy in rodent models of RA and septic shock.

There are many p38 kinase inhibitors in clinical development and the first human trials have began. These orally bioavailable agents have the potential to modulate inducible expression of pro-inflammatory cytokines.

Interleukin-1β converting enzyme (ICE) inhibition

Inhibition of interleukin-1β converting enzyme (ICE or caspase-1) offers a potential means to treat autoimmune diseases. Pro-IL-1β is synthesized by activated monocytes and macrophages as a biologically inactive precursor. ICE is a cysteine protease that catalyzes the conversion of the inactive precursor form of IL-1β into a biologically active mature form. IL-1β mediates inflammatory responses, regulates Fas-mediated apoptosis of lymphoid cells, and is believed to be involved in the progression of RA.

In animal models, ICE inhibition slows progression of disease, and mouse knockout models for ICE do not develop CIA. VE-13045, an ICE inhibitor, reduced severity of CIA when given prophylactically or following disease onset [35]. Synthetic ICE inhibitors are under investigation for the treatment of human RA.

Complement inhibition

Upon activation of the complement system, C5 is cleaved into its pro-inflammatory components C5a and C5b-9. These activated components act as pro-inflammatory mediators leading to leukocyte activation, cytokine release, production of matrix metalloproteinases and up-regulation of adhesion molecules. With the use of anti-C5 antibodies it is possible to prevent selectively the cleavage of C5 into its byproducts, whilst preserving the body's normal abilities to generate C3b and to maintain opsonization and immune complex functions.

In murine models of CIA, antibodies to C5 demonstrated substantially the ability to prevent the development of arthritis, as well as to reduce arthritis in animals with established disease [36]. The results of a Phase I study examining a humanized anti-CD5 antibody (h5G1.1) in RA showed that administration of a single dose of the agent was generally well tolerated [37]. In the 8 mg/kg cohort there was a suggestion of improvement in the number of tender and swollen joints as well as a significant reduction in the mean CRP levels. A Phase II multi-dose safety and efficacy study of h5G1.1 in RA patients is in progess.

Matrix metalloproteinase inhibition

Therapeutic agents are being developed to inhibit the enzymes responsible for the destruction of cartilage and bone. Several types of proteases are involved in connective tissue degradation, including matrix metalloproteinases (MMPs), aspartic proteases, cysteine proteases and serine proteases [1]. The MMPs considered to be of the greatest importance in the development of tissue damage in arthritis are listed in Table 1 and include members of the collagenase, gelatinase and stromelysin families.

MMPs are constitutively expressed at low levels. Following the appropriate stimulus, MMPs are inducibly expressed and activated by synoviocytes and macrophages. Stimuli include: cytokines (IL-1, IL-10, TNF-α), platelet derived growth factor (PDGF), bacterial toxins, cell-cell interactions, iron, serum amyloid A-like protein and β_2-microglobulin-like-protein [1]. These proteases result in cartilage and connective tissue degradation. There are naturally occurring inhibitors of MMPs (e.g. α_2-macroglobulin, TGF-β, all-trans-retinoic acid and tissue inhibitors of metalloproteinase [TIMP]). These molecules may help maintain the balance between catabolic and anabolic activity within connective tissue structures.

There are two options for pharmacological intervention aimed at inhibiting MMPs:

1. to augment production of the naturally occurring MMP inhibitors (MMPIs)

2. to deliver synthetic versions of selective-MMP inhibitors

In a more practical sense the anthracycline family of antibiotics, and in particular minocycline, have been shown to be of utility in the treatment of RA [38-40]. While not completely understood, the efficacy of these antibiotics as therapy for RA is believed to be related to the inhibition of MMPs (MMP 1,2,12,13) [41].

Table 1. Matrix metalloproteinases with the greatest likelihood of involvement in the development of arthritis.

MMP-1	Interstitial collagenase
MMP-2	Gelatinase/type IV collagenase
MMP-3	Stromelysin 1
MMP-8	Neutrophil collagenase
MMP-9	Gelatinase/type V collagenase
MMP-13	Interstitial collagenase

Adapted from Harris ED, editor. Rheumatoid Arthritis. Philadelphia: Saunders WB, 1997 [1].

Doxycycline is believed to inhibit MMPs more effectively than other members of the tetracycline family. It has subsequently been studied as an intravenous therapy in two unsuccessful short-term studies for the treatment of RA [42,43].

Synthetic agents specifically designed to inhibit MMPs have been developed for study in the treatment of RA and osteoarthritis (OA). It is hoped that these will have better efficacy and possibly fewer side effects. Many compounds have been utilized in studies thus far, but few data have been published to date. BAY 12-9566, a known inhibitor of MMP-2, 3, 8, 9 and 13, has been shown to prevent the breakdown of cartilage *in vitro* and in animal models of OA. It has been studied in 35 patients with OA scheduled for elective total knee replacement. A possible beneficial effect was found in one dose cohort with statistically significant decreases in denatured collagen and increases in total collagen. However, no observations were made on clinical impact [44]. While these findings have led to optimism that MMP inhibitors might have a beneficial effect on cartilage metabolism *in vivo*, investigation with BAY 12-9566 was halted in September 1999. Investigators in a cancer trial had reported decreased survival times in patients receiving BAY 12-9566 compared to those receiving placebo. It is uncertain what implications these findings will have on the study of other MMP inhibitors.

Questions remain about the ability to demonstrate that MMPIs have utility in the treatment of RA. The outcome tools currently being utilized may not be sufficiently sensitive or specific enough to demonstrate prevention of structural decline, or improvement in structure. Also, given the relatively downstream point of intervention with MMPIs, it is uncertain whether these agents will have a significant impact on pain, swelling or function.

Tremendous progress, tremendous potential

Over the past decade, tremendous progress has been made towards a better understanding of the underlying pathophysiology of RA. Based on this knowledge, novel therapeutic agents, such as TNF-α antagonists, have been developed, demonstrated to have efficacy in clinical trials and implemented in clinical practice. Although such agents have great clinical value, they are in no manner curative. With the start of the new millennium the next generation of novel biological agents, designed to induce immune tolerance at a fundamental level, are undergoing thorough evaluation in human clinical trials. Of critical importance is clear demonstration of the safety and efficacy of novel therapeutic agents in human patients. There is frequent discordance between data generated from animal models as compared with human patients. An air of skepticism will be crucial in the interpretation of animal data and its applicability to humans having what are believed to be similar diseases.

References

1. Harris ED, editor. Rheumatoid Arthritis. Philadelphia: WB Saunders, 1997.
2. Kavanaugh A, Paulus H, Olsen N et al. Allele- and antigen-specific treatment of rheumatoid arthritis: a double blind, placebo controlled phase I trial. Arthritis Rheum 1999; [abstract #43].
3. Kivitz A, Paulus H, Olsen N et al. Allele- and antigen-specific treatment of rheumatoid arthritis: a double blind, placebo controlled phase I trial. (Submitted for publication).
4. Moreland LW, Morgan EE, Adamson TC et al. T cell receptor peptide vaccination in rheumatoid arthritis: a placebo-controlled trial using a combination of Vβ3, Vβ14 and Vβ17 peptides. Arthritis Rheum 1998;41(11):1919–29.

5. Matsumoto AK, Moreland LW, Strand V et al. Results of phase IIb rheumatoid arthritis clinical trial using T cell receptor peptides. Arthritis Rheum 1999; [abstract #281].

6. Butler DM, Malfait AM, Mason LJ et al. DBA/1 mice expressing the human TNF-α transgene develop a severe, erosive arthritis: characterization of the cytokine cascade and cellular composition. J Immunol 1997;159:2867–76.

7. McIntyre KW, Shuster DJ, Gillooly KM et al. Reduced incidence and severity of collagen-induced arthritis in IL-12-deficient mice. Eur J Immunol 1996;26:2933–8.

8. Matthys P, Vermeire K, Mitera T et al. Anti-IL-12 antibody prevents the development and progression of collagen-induced arthritis in IFN-γ receptor-deficient mice. Eur J Immunol 1998;28:2143–51.

9. Butler DM, Malfait AM, Maini RN et al. Anti-IL-12 and anti-TNF antibodies synergistically suppress the progression of murine collagen-induced arthritis. Eur J Immunol 1999;29:2205–12.

10. Kim WU, Min SY, Cho ML et al. The role of IL-12 in inflammatory activity of patients with rheumatoid arthritis (RA). Clin Exp Immunol 2000;119(1):175–81.

11. Peeva E, Fishman AD, Goddard G et al. Rheumatoid arthritis exacerbation caused by exogenous IL-12. Arthritis Rheum 2000;43:461–3.

12. Berner B, Akca D, Jung T et al. Analysis of Th1 and Th2 cytokines expressing CD4+ and CD8+ T cells in rheumatoid arthritis by flow cytometry. J Rheumatol 2000;27:1128–35.

13. IFNb Multiple Sclerosis Study Group. Interferon β-1b is effective in relapsing-remitting multiple sclerosis. I. Clinical results of a multicenter, randomized, double-blind, placebo-controlled trial. Neurology 1993;43:655–61.

14. Smeets TJ, Dayer JM, Kraan MC et al. The effects of interferon-β treatment of synovial inflammation and expression of metalloproteinases in patients with rheumatoid arthritis. Arthritis Rheum 2000;43:270–4.

15. Hirano T, Matsuda T, Turner M et al. Excessive production of interleukin 6/B cell stimulatory factor-2 in rheumatoid arthritis. Eur J Immunol 1988;18:1797–801.

16. Brozik M, Rosztoczy I, Meretey K et al. Interleukin 6 levels in synovial fluids of patients with different arthritides: correlation with local IgM rheumatoid factor and systemic acute phase protein production. J Rheumatol 1992;19:63–8.

17. Uson J, Balsa A, Pascual-Salcedo D et al. Soluble interleukin 6 (IL-6) receptor and IL-6 levels in serum and synovial fluid of patients with different arthropathies. J Rheumatol 1997;24:2069–75.

18. Wendling D, Racadot E, Wijdenes J. Treatment of severe rheumatoid arthritis by anti-interleukin 6 monoclonal antibody. J Rheumatol 1993;20:259–62.

19. Panayi GS. Targeting of cells involved in the pathogenesis of rheumatoid arthritis. Rheumatology 1999;38(Suppl. 2):8–10.

20. Durie FH, Fava RA, Foy TM et al. Prevention of collagen-induced arthritis with an antibody to gp39, the ligand for CD40. Science 1993;261:1328–30.

21. Sekine C, Yagita H, Miyasaka N et al. Expression and function of CD40 in rheumatoid arthritis synovium. J Rheumatol 1998;25:1048–53.

22. Shimoyama Y, Nagafuchi H, Suzuki N et al. Synovium infiltrating T cells induce excessive synovial cell function through CD28/B7 pathway in patients with rheumatoid arthritis. J Rheumatol 1999;26:2094–101.

23. Liu MF, Kohsaka H, Sakurai H et al. The presence of costimulatory molecules CD86 and CD28 in rheumatoid arthritis synovium. Arthritis Rheum 1996;39:110–4.

24. Balsa A, Dixey J, Sansom DM et al. Differential expression of the costimulatory molecules B7.1 (CD80) and B7.2 (CD86) in rheumatoid synovial tissue. Br J Rheumatol 1996;35:33–7.

25. Ranheim EA, Kipps TJ. Elevated expression of CD80 (B7/BB1) and other accessory molecules on synovial fluid mononuclear cell subsets in rheumatoid arthritis. Arthritis Rheum 1994;37:1637–46.

26. Webb LM, Walmsley MJ, Feldmann M. Prevention and amelioration of collagen-induced arthritis by blockade of the CD28 co-stimulatory pathway: requirement for both B7-1 and B7-2. Eur J Immunol 1996;26:2320–8.

27. Schwartz RS. The new immunology—the end of immunosuppressive drug therapy? N Engl J Med 1999;340:1754–6.

28. Knoerzer DB, Karr RW, Schwartz BD et al. Collagen-induced arthritis in the BB rat. Prevention of disease by treatment with CTLA-4-Ig. J Clin Invest 1995;96:987–93.

29. Abrams JR, Lebwohl MG, Guzzo CA et al. CTLA-4-Ig-mediated blockade of T cell costimulation in patients with psoriasis vulgaris. J Clin Invest 1999;103:1243–52.

30. Evans CH, Robbins PD, Ghivizzani SC et al. Clinical trial to assess the safety, feasibility, and efficacy of transferring a potentially anti-arthritic cytokine gene to human joints with rheumatoid arthritis. Hum Gene Ther 1996;7:1261–80.

31. Evans CH, Robbins PD, Ghivizzani SC et al. Results from the first human clinical trial of gene therapy for arthritis. Arthritis Rheum 1999; [abstract #600].

32. Evans CH, Ghivizzani SC, Kang R et al. Gene therapy for rheumatic diseases. Arthritis Rheum 1999;42:1–16.

33. Commander H. Biotechnology industry responds to gene therapy death. Nat Med 2000;6:118.

34. Tibbles LA, Woodgett JR. The stress-activated protein kinase pathways. Cell Mol Life Sci 1999;55:1230–54.

35. Ku G, Faust T, Lauffer LL et al. Interleukin-1β converting enzyme inhibition blocks progression of type II collagen-induced arthritis in mice. Cytokine 1996;8:377–86.

36. Wang Y, Rollins SA, Madri JA et al. Anti-C5 monoclonal antibody therapy prevents collagen-induced arthritis and ameliorates established disease. Proc Natl Acad Sci USA 1995;92:8955–9.

37. Jain RI, Moreland LW, Caldwell JR et al. A single dose, placebo controlled, double blind, phase I study of the humanized anti-C5 antibody H5g1.1 in patients with rheumatoid arthritis. Arthritis Rheum 1999; [abstract #42].

38. Kloppenburg M, Breedveld FC, Terwiel JP et al. Minocycline in active rheumatoid arthritis: a double-blind, placebo-controlled trial. Arthritis Rheum 1994;37:629–36.

39. Tilley BC, Alarcon GS, Heyse SP et al. Minocycline in rheumatoid arthritis. A 48-week, double-blind, placebo-controlled trial. Ann Intern Med 1995;122:81–9.

40. O'Dell JR, Haire CE, Palmer W et al. Treatment of early rheumatoid arthritis with minocycline or placebo: results of a randomized, double-blind, placebo-controlled trial. Arthritis Rheum 1997;40:842–8.

41. Furst DE. Leflunomide, mycophenolic acid and matrix metalloproteinase inhibitors. Rheumatology 1999;38(Suppl. 2):14–8.

42. Pillemer S, Gulko P, Ligier S et al. Pilot clinical trial of intravenous doxycycline versus placebo for rheumatoid arthritis (RA). Arthritis Rheum 1999; [abstract #61].

43. St.Clair EW, Wilkinson WE, Drew R et al. Intravenous doxycycline therapy in rheumatoid arthritis (RA): a randomized, placebo-controlled pilot trial. Arthritis Rheum 1999; [abstract #1033].

44. Leff RL, Elias I, Ionescu M et al. Molecular changes in human osteoarthritic cartilage after three weeks of oral administration of Bay 12-9566, a novel matrix metalloproteinase inhibitor. Arthritis Rheum 1999; [abstract #1997].

i

Index